Vitamin C
the Common Cold
and the Flu

Vitamin C
the Common Cold
and the Flu

LINUS PAULING

W. H. FREEMAN AND COMPANY
San Francisco

Library of Congress Cataloging in Publication Data

Pauling, Linus Carl, 1901-
  Vitamin C, the common cold, and the flu.

  Bibliography: p.
  Includes index.
  1. Vitamin C—Therapeutic use. 2. Cold
(Disease)—Prevention. 3. Influenza—Prevention.
  I. Title.
  RM666.A79P32   616.2′05′061   76-28516
  ISBN 0-7167-0360-2
  ISBN 0-7167-0361-0 pbk.

Printed in the United States of America

1 2 3 4 5 6 7 8 9

TO

AVA HELEN PAULING

Contents

Preface

Six years ago many people were already convinced, on the basis of their own experience, that an increased intake of vitamin C provides some protection against the common cold, even though most physicians and authorities in the field of nutrition continued to describe vitamin C as having no value in controlling the common cold or any other disease except its specific deficiency disease, scurvy. When I examined the medical literature I found that a number of excellent studies had been carried out, and that most of them showed that vitamin C does have value in controlling the common cold. My concern about the failure of the medical authorities to pay the deserved attention to the existing evidence caused me to write my book *Vitamin C and the Common Cold,* which was published in 1970 and has been translated into many foreign languages.

When this book was published it received favorable comments from some reviewers, but was quite strongly criticized by others. The discussion that followed stimulated a number of investigators, including Professor George Beaton, head of the Department of Nutriton in the School of Hygiene of the University of Toronto, to begin controlled trials. These trials all supported the conclusion that vitamin C has value in controlling the common cold. As a result, the medical and nutritional authorities no longer claim that vitamin C has no value in connection with the common cold, although they may contend that the amount of protection provided by it is not great enough to justify the bother and expense of taking the vitamin.

In the course of my continued studies of vitamin C, I learned that this vitamin exerts a general antiviral action and provides some protection not only against the common cold but also against other viral diseases, including influenza. The common cold is a nuisance, but is not very dangerous. Only rarely does it lead to complications that cause death. Influenza (the flu), on the other hand, is a very serious and dangerous disease. In the great influenza pandemic of 1918–1919 the disease was contracted by about 85 percent of the population in all countries and killed about 1 percent, including many healthy young adults—the estimated total number of deaths being about 20 million. An outbreak of influenza in early 1976 with a virus similar to that of the 1918–1919 pandemic has recently caused great concern. The President of the United States announced that the government would subsidize a program costing over $135,000,000 for preparation of vaccine that might permit the epidemic expected in the 1976–1977 winter to be controlled. Little mention has been made, however, of the value of vitamin C in protecting against influenza. In this book I present a discussion of the evidence about vitamin C and influenza, and also bring the discussion of the common cold up to date. I hope that the book will help many people to avoid serious illness and will enable them to lead healthier and longer lives. For their help in the preparation of this book I thank Dr. Linus Pauling, Jr., Professor Crellin Pauling, Dr. Arthur B. Robinson, Brian Leibovitz, and Mrs. Dorothy Munro. I continue to be grateful to Albert Szent-Györgyi for having isolated L-ascorbic acid for the first time a half century ago and Irwin Stone for having aroused my interest in it a decade ago.

Linus Pauling

LINUS PAULING INSTITUTE OF SCIENCE AND MEDICINE
2700 SAND HILL ROAD
MENLO PARK, CALIFORNIA 94025

31 July 1976

Vitamin C
the Common Cold
and the Flu

Introduction

The idea that I should write a book about vitamin C began to develop in my mind about ten years ago. In April 1966 I received a letter from Irwin Stone, a biochemist whom I had met at the Carl Neuberg Medal Award dinner in New York the previous month. He mentioned in his letter that I had expressed a desire to live for the next fifteen or twenty years. He said that he would like to see me remain in good health for the next *fifty* years, and that he was accordingly sending me a description of his high-level ascorbic-acid* regimen, which he had developed during the preceding three decades. My wife and I began the regimen recommended by Stone. We noticed an increased feeling of wellbeing, and especially a striking decrease in the number of colds that we caught, and in their severity.

---

*In this book the terms "ascorbic acid" and "vitamin C" are used interchangeably (see Chapter 4).

In the introduction to my book *Vitamin C and the Common Cold* (1970) I made the following statement at this point:

> Dr. Stone was, of course, exaggerating. I estimate that complete control of the common cold and associated disorders would increase the average life expectancy by two or three years. The improvement in the general state of health resulting from ingesting the optimum amount of ascorbic acid might lead to an equal additional increase in life expectancy.

It is my opinion now, after an additional six years of study in this field, that for most people the improvement in health associated with the ingestion of the optimum amount of ascorbic aid is not just such as to lead to an increase in life expectancy by only four to six years; instead, my present estimate is that the increase probably lies in the range twelve to eighteen years. Some of the reasons for this estimate are given in the following chapters of this book.

During the period from 1966 to 1970 I gradually became aware of the existence of an extraordinary contradiction between the opinions of different people about the value of vitamin C in preventing and ameliorating the common cold. Many people believe that vitamin C helps prevent colds; on the other hand, most physicians at that time denied that this vitamin has much value in treating the common cold. For example, in the discussion of the treatment of the common cold in his excellent book *Health* (1970) Dr. Benjamin A Kogan made the following statement: "Research has shown that vitamin C, in the form of fruit juice, however pleasant, is useless in preventing or shortening colds." Dr. John M. Adams did not mention vitamin C in his book *Viruses and Colds: the Modern Plague* (1967). More recent books by physicians contain statements such as the following: "I would again, however, like to stress that there is no evidence to support the contention that vitamin C prevents the common cold and only shaky evidence to suggest that it may lessen the effects of colds" (Johnson, 1975).

The difference of opinion was brought sharply to my attention by the publication of an article about vitamin C in the magazine *Mademoiselle* in November 1969. I was quoted as supporting the use of large amounts of vitamin C. Dr. Fredrick J. Stare, described as "one of the country's Big Names in nutrition," was quoted as saying "Vitamin C and colds—that was disproved twenty years ago. I'll tell you about just one very careful study. Of five thousand students at the University of Minnesota, half were given large doses of C, half a placebo. Their medical histories were followed for two years—and no difference was found in the frequency, severity, or duration of their colds. And yes, stores of C are depleted in massive, lingering infection—not in week-long colds."

The study to which Dr. Stare was referring had been carried out by Cowan, Diehl, and Baker; the article describing their results was published in 1942 (see Chapter 6). When I read this article I found that the study involved only about four hundred students, rather than five thousand, that it was continued for half a year, not two years, and that it involved use of only 200 milligrams of vitamin C per day, which is not a large dose. Moreover, the investigators reported that the students receiving the vitamin C had 31 percent fewer days of illness per subject.

The fact that Dr. Stare, as well as the investigators themselves (Cowan, Diehl, and Baker), had not considered a decrease by 31 percent in the days of illness as important suggested to me that an examination of the medical literature might provide more information about this matter. The August 1967 issue of the journal *Nutrition Reviews* contained a brief editorial article about vitamin C and the common cold, in which a number of articles on the subject were mentioned. Dr. Stare, who is a professor in the Department of Nutrition of the School of Public Health of Harvard University, was editor of this journal at that time. The conclusion reported in this article was that "there is no conclusive evidence that ascorbic acid has any protective effect against, or any therapeutic effect on, the course of the common cold in healthy people not depleted of ascorbic acid. There is also no evidence for a general antiviral, or symptomatic prophylactic effect of ascorbic acid."

I examined the reports mentioned in this editorial article (they are all discussed in Chapter 6 and Appendix III), and found that my own conclusions, on the basis of the studies themselves, were different from those expressed in the editorial article.

We may ask why the physicians and authorities on nutrition have remained so lacking in enthusiasm about a substance that was reported three decades ago to decrease the illness with colds by 31 percent, when taken regularly in rather small daily amounts. I surmise that several factors have contributed to this lack of enthusiasm. In the search for a drug to combat a disease the effort is usually made to find one that is 100 percent effective. (I must say that I do not understand, however, why Cowan, Diehl, and Baker did not repeat their study with use of larger amounts of vitamin C per day.) Also, there seems to have existed a feeling that the intake of vitamin C should be kept as small as possible, even though this vitamin is known to have extremely low toxicity. This attitude is, of course, proper for *drugs*—substances not normally present in the human body and almost always rather highly toxic—but it does not apply to ascorbic acid. Another factor has probably been the lack of interest of the drug companies in a natural substance that is available at a low price and cannot be patented.

Irwin Stone's letter to me came at a time in my own development when it was possible for me to contribute to the subject. For many years, since 1935, I had been working on the general problem of the relation between physiological activity and molecular structure of the substances present in the human body. With my students and colleagues I had worked on the structure of the complex molecules of hemoglobin and other proteins, on the nature of antibodies (which provide a natural protection against infectious disease), on the nature of sickle-cell anemia and other molecular diseases, and, beginning in 1954, on the possibility that mental diseases often have a molecular basis. In the course of these investigations I became interested in the vitamins, and I learned that Dr. A. Hoffer and Dr. H. Osmond had begun treating schizophrenic patients with large doses of a vitamin, either niacin or niacinamide. I was astonished to read that they recommended the use of between 3 grams and 18 grams of niacin or niacinamide per day in the treatment of schizophrenia. This amount is hundreds of times as much as is needed to prevent the dietary deficiency disease pellagra. I had formulated some ideas about why, for some people, at any rate, improved health might result from an increase in intake of certain vitamins, and later on, in 1968, I published these ideas (see Chapter 9). Stone's letter, together with some studies by other people, and those by my colleague Arthur B. Robinson and me on ascorbic acid in relation to schizophrenia were significant in encouraging me to examine the matter of vitamin C and the common cold, as described in my 1970 book and in this book.

The common cold and influenza are infections by viruses that circulate throughout the world. They rapidly die out in a small isolated population. If the incidence of colds and influenza could be decreased enough throughout the world these diseases would disappear, as smallpox has in the British Isles. I foresee the achievement of this goal, perhaps within a decade or two, in some parts of the world. Some period of quarantine of travelers might be needed, so long as a major part of the world's people are poverty stricken and especially subject to infectious diseases because of malnutrition, including lack of ascorbic acid in the proper amount.

To achieve this goal a change in the attitude of the public and of the patient may be required. A person with the cold or the flu should feel that he should isolate himself, in order not to spread the virus to other people, and social pressure should operate on him to help him to act in such a way as not to harm others. We have recently experienced a change in feeling about the "right" of cigarette smokers to pollute the atmosphere and distress non-smokers. A similar change in feeling about the "right" of a person to spread his viruses and infect other people, so long as he himself is able to stagger about, would benefit the world.

1

The Common Cold

The common cold causes a tremendous amount of human suffering. The average incidence of colds is about three per person per year. A cold usually lasts from three to ten days. During part of this period the victim may feel miserable. If he is wise, he spends a few days in bed. The cold may be followed by serious complications—bronchitis, sinus infection, infection of the middle ear, infection of the mastoid bone (mastoiditis), meningitis, bronchopneumonia or lobar pneumonia, or exacerbation of some other disease, such as arthritis or kidney disease or heart disease.

The common cold (acute coryza) is an inflammation of the upper respiratory tract caused by infection with a virus.* This

---

*A discussion of the many viruses that can cause the common cold is given in the book *The Common Cold,* by Sir Christopher Andrewes, 1965. (Note that full bibliographic information is given for all references, listed alphabetically by name of the first author, beginning on page 199.)

infection alters the physiology of the mucous membrane of the nose, the paranasal sinuses, and the throat. The common cold occurs more often than all other diseases combined. The common cold does not occur in small isolated communities. Exposure to the virus, carried by other persons, is needed. For example, the Norwegian island of Spitsbergen used to be isolated during seven months of the year. The 507 residents of the principal town of the island, Longyear, were nearly free of colds through the cold winter, with only four colds recorded in three months. Then within two weeks after the arrival of the first ship some two hundred of the residents had become ill with colds (Paul and Freese, 1933).

Development of a cold after exposure to the virus is determined to some extent by the state of health of the person and by environmental factors. Fatigue, chilling of the body, wearing of wet clothing and wet shoes, and the presence of irritating substances in the air make it more likely that the cold will develop. Experimental studies indicate, however, that these factors are not so important as is generally believed (Andrewes, 1965; Debré and Celers, 1970, page 539). The period of incubation, between exposure and the manifestation of symptoms, is usually two or three days. The first symptoms are a feeling of roughness or soreness of the throat, development of a nasal discharge, attacks of sneezing, and a sensation of fullness and irritation in the upper respiratory tract. Headache, general malaise (an indefinite feeling of uneasiness or discomfort), and chills (a sensation of coldness attended with convulsive shaking of the body, pinched face, pale skin, and blue lips) are often present. A slight increase in temperature, usually to not over 101°F (38.3°C), may occur. The mucous membranes of the nose and pharynx are swollen. One nostril or both nostrils may be blocked by the thickened secretions. The skin around the nostrils may become sore, and cold sores (caused by the virus *Herpes simplex*) may develop on the lips.

The customary treatment for the common cold includes resting in bed, drinking fruit juice or water, ingesting a simple and nutritious diet, preventing irritants such as tobacco smoke from entering the respiratory tract, and alleviating the symptoms to some extent by the use of aspirin, phenacetin, antihistamines, and other drugs (see Chapter 13). After some days the tissues of the nose and throat, weakened by the virus infection, often are invaded by bacteria. This secondary infection may cause the nasal secretions to become purulent (to contain pus). Also, the secondary infection may spread to the sinuses, the middle ears, the tonsils, the pharynx, the larynx, the trachea, the bronchi, and the lungs. As mentioned above, mastoiditis, meningitis, and other serious infections may follow. Control of the common cold thus would lead to a decrease in the incidence of more serious diseases.

Not everyone is susceptible to infection with the common cold. Most investigators have noted that an appreciable proportion of the population, 6 to 10 percent, never have colds. This fact provides justification for hope that a significant decrease in the number of colds can be achieved through increase in the resistance of individuals to viral infection. It is likely that the ability of 6 to 10 percent of the population to avoid colds is the result of their natural powers of resistance. Like other physiological properties, the resistance of individuals to viral infection probably can be represented by a distribution curve that has approximately the normal bell shape. The 6 to 10 percent of the population that are resistant to colds presumably correspond to the tail end of the curve, those people with the largest natural powers of resisting viral infections. If in some way the natural resistance of the whole population could be shifted upward, a larger percentage of the population would lie in the range corresponding to complete resistance to the infection, and would never have colds. This argument indicates strongly that a study of the factors involved in the natural resistance to viral infection, such as nutritional factors, could lead to a significant decrease in the susceptibility of the population as a whole to the common cold. (See, for example, Debré and Celers, 1970, page 539.)

I have made a rough estimate of the significance of the common cold, measured in dollars. Let us assume that the average loss of time because of serious illness with the common cold is seven days per person per year. The person suffering from a cold or series of colds during the year might stay away from work, or he might have a decreased effectiveness, or might be sufficiently ill to feel that the seven days are wasted, because of feeling miserable. In any case, a measure of the damage done by the common cold might be roughly taken as his loss of productivity and income for the seven days during the year when he is most seriously ill. The personal income of the people of the United States is about 800 billion dollars per year. The income per week is this quantity divided by fifty two, which is about 15 billion dollars. We may accordingly be justified in saying that the damage done by the common cold to the people of the United States each year can be described roughly as corresponding to a monetary loss of 15 billion dollars per year.*

---

*A somewhat smaller estimate, 5 billion dollars per year, was given by Fabricant and Conklin in their book *The Dangerous Cold,* 1965.

This estimate corresponds to a loss in income or its equivalent in wellbeing of about seventy-five dollars per year per person in the United States.

It is easy to understand why the people of the United States spend hundreds of millions of dollars per year on cold medicines, despite their limited effectiveness, in an effort to reduce their physical discomfort and loss of income.

In the medical literature it is usually said that no clearly effective method of treatment of the common cold has been developed. The various drugs that are prescribed or recommended have some value in making the patient more comfortable, by giving him relief from some of the more distressing symptoms, but they have little effect on the duration of the cold. I believe, on the other hand, that most colds can be prevented or largely ameliorated by control of the diet, without the use of any drugs. The dietary substance that is involved is vitamin C, which is known to be the substance ascorbic acid.**

Ascorbic acid is a food. It is, in fact, an essential food for all human beings. It is present, in greater or smaller amounts, in many ordinary foodstuffs, including fruits, vegetables, and meats. For about forty years it has been available in pure form, either separated from a fruit or vegetable in which it occurs or made from a sugar (glucose or sorbose) by a simple chemical reaction, similar to the chemical reactions that take place continually in living plants and animals.

A person's health depends in part on the foods that he eats. Certain amounts of some foods are needed for life. These

---

**As noted in the Introduction, the words "ascorbic acid" and "vitamin C" are used interchangeably. I have retained use of the term "vitamin C" in order to emphasize the role of ascorbic acid as an essential nutrient, "ascorbic acid" to call attention to its existence as a pure substance.

essential foods include the essential amino acids, essential fats, certain minerals, and the various vitamins, including vitamin C.

A person who eats no vitamin C will become sick in a few months, even though his diet is adequate in other respects, and then die. A small intake of vitamin C, which for many people may lie somewhere within the range 5 mg (milligrams) to 15 mg per day, is enough to prevent a human being from dying of vitamin C deficiency, which is called scurvy. The amount that keeps him from dying of scurvy may not, however, be the amount that puts him in the best of health. The amount that puts him in the best of health, which may be called the optimum amount, is not reliably known; but there is some evidence that for different people it lies in the range between 250 mg and 10,000 mg per day; that is, between ¼ g (gram) and 10 g per day.*

The evidence indicating the need for these larger amounts of vitamin C in order to achieve the best of health, including protection against the common cold, is presented in later chapters in this book. The discussion of the optimum intake of vitamin C for averting and ameliorating the common cold and influenza is given in Chapters 6, 7, and 14.

The relatively low cost of dietary control of the common cold, in comparison with the monetary equivalent of the damage done by the disease and the large amounts of money now spent on ineffective medicines, is discussed in Chapter 14. Advice about how to buy vitamin C is given in Appendix I, and a rather small amount of information about other vitamins is given in Appendix II.

---

*One pound equals 453.6 g, and one ounce equals 28.35 g. One kilogram equals 2.2 pounds. A level teaspoon of ascorbic acid is 4.4 g.

It is pointed out near the end of Chapter 2 that heart disease is the principal cause of death in the United States, with cancer second, cerebrovascular disease third, and influenza and pneumonia fourth. Essentially no deaths are attributed to the common cold, although the weakening effect of an upper respiratory viral infection may sometimes lead to death from a secondary bacterial infection or some other disease. The value of a proper intake of vitamin C goes far beyond its effectiveness in decreasing the amount of suffering with the common cold. There is a continually increasing body of evidence that the optimum intake of vitamin C decreases both the morbidity and mortality with heart disease, cerebrovascular disease, and cancer, as well as infectious diseases in general. Some of this evidence is presented in Appendix IV. It is pointed out there that vitamin C is not a wonder drug, a drug that cures a particular disease. It is instead a substance required for the effective operation of many of the essential biochemical and physiological processes that take place in our bodies, and especially of the various mechanisms that protect us against the agents of disease. The amount of protection against disease and death that is provided by the optimum intake of vitamin C is not yet known. No epidemiological study of the effect of a large intake of vitamin C on the general health of human beings has been made. That the effect is a great one is indicated by the results of a study of death rates of older people reported by Chope and Breslow (1956). The most pronounced correlation that they found between any environmental, behavioral, or nutritional factor and the age-corrected death rate was the one with vitamin C; the subjects with a low intake of vitamin C had 2.5 times the chance of death at a given age as those with a high intake. (This study is discussed in greater detail in Chapter 10.)

It is, of course, essential that everyone consult his physician in case of serious illness. An improved diet should improve your general health; but you cannot hope that it will protect you completely from "the rotten diseases of the south, the guts-griping, ruptures, catarrhs, loads o' gravel i' the back, lethargies, cold palsies, raw eyes, dirt-rotten livers, wheezing lungs, bladders full of imposthume, sciaticas, limekilns i' the palm, incurable boneache, and the riveled fee-simple of the tetter" (Shakespeare, *Troilus and Cressida*). Nevertheless, an increased intake of vitamin C and some other nutritional measures may be of tremendous value to you when illness strikes.

2

Influenza

Influenza is a highly contagious disease characterized by fever, aches and pains, prostration, and inflammation of the respiratory mucous membranes. It is not the same disease as the common cold, although some of the signs and symptoms, such as increased nasal secretion, are similar. Influenza, like the common cold, is caused by a virus, but the influenza viruses belong to a different family from the cold viruses and the two diseases manifest themselves in some significantly different ways.

The incubation time for influenza (time from exposure to onset of symptoms) is short—about two days. The onset usually is sudden. It is marked by chills, fever, headache, lassitude and general malaise, anorexia (loss of appetite), muscular aches and pains, and sometimes nausea, occasionally with vomiting. Respiratory symptoms, such as sneezing and nasal discharge, may be present, but are usually less pronounced than with the common cold. Coughing, without production of sputum, may occur, and hoarseness sometimes develops. The fever usually lasts for two to four days. In mild cases the temperature reaches 101° to 103° F (38.3° to 39.4° C) and in severe cases as much as 105° F (40.6° C).

Treatment consists of rest in bed, continuing for twenty-four to forty-eight hours after the temperature has become normal. Antibiotics may be used to control secondary bacterial infections. The diet should be light, with a large intake (3,000 to 3,500 ml per day—about 7 pints) of water and fruit juices. Except during a pandemic, almost all of the patients recover completely.

Influenza is an old disease. Hippocrates in his book *Epidemics* described a disease raging at Perinthos in Crete about 400 B.C., in such a way as to permit its identification as influenza. An influenza epidemic (occurrence of the disease in many people in a community) was reported in 1557–1558 and a pandemic (occurrence in most of the people in a country or several countries) spread throughout Europe in 1580–1581. Other epidemics or pandemics broke out in 1658, 1676, 1732–1733, 1837, 1889–1890, 1918–1919, 1933, and 1957, and it is feared that one may occur in 1976–1977 or 1977–1978.

The most serious influenza pandemic was that of 1918–1919. It swept over the whole world in three successive waves, May to July 1918, September to December 1918, and March to May 1919. It is thought to have arisen in Spain, and it was popularly called the Spanish flu (Collier, 1974). It broke out almost simultaneously in all the European nations, and probably was rapidly spread because of the movement of troops and because of wartime conditions. The first wave did not reach some parts of the world, including South America, Australia, and many islands in the Atlantic and Pacific Oceans. The second wave, which caused most of the deaths, covered the whole world except the islands St. Helena and Mauritius. Between 80 and 90 percent of the people in most countries contracted the disease, and about 20 million died. The disease was clearly not the same as ordinary influenza, because in 1918–1919 most of the deaths occurred among young people, whereas in the preceding and following years most of the deaths from influenza were among the old.

THE INFLUENZA VIRUSES

From 1892 to 1918 it was thought that influenza was caused by a bacterium, called Pfeiffer's bacillus, that had been isolated from sputum or blood of influenza patients. Then in 1918 the French investigator Debré observed a similarity in the immune response of patients with influenza to those with measles, a viral disease, and concluded that influenza was probably also caused by a virus. Proof of this suggestion was immediately reported by Selter (1918) in Germany, Nicolle and Lebailly (1918) in Tunis, and Dujarric de la Rivière (1918) in France. The proof was obtained by forcing infected sputum and blood through a filter with pores so fine that no bacteria could pass through them. It was found that the filtered liquid put in the nasal passages of monkeys and of human volunteers caused them to develop the disease, which was accordingly ascribed to a virus, the particles of which are much smaller than bacteria.

Isolation of strains of influenza virus, permitting thorough studies of their properties to be made, was achieved in 1933 by the British investigators Smith, Andrewes, and Laidlaw. An account of the way in which this important step was taken has been published by Christopher Andrewes (1965). During the influenza epidemic of 1933 Andrewes and Wilson Smith of the British National Institute for Medical Research were working on influenza when Andrewes became ill with the disease. Smith had him gargle with salt water and used the solution in an attempt to infect rabbits, guinea pigs, mice, hedgehogs, hamsters, and monkeys, but without success. Patrick Laidlaw, in the same Institute, had been able to infect ferrets with dog distemper; he found that the Andrewes garglings introduced into the noses of ferrets caused them to become ill with the flu. Later a way was found to infect mice with influenza.

In fact, there had for a long time been evidence that some strains of influenza virus infect certain animals, as well as human beings. Observers had noted that in the 1732 epidemic horses seemed to be suffering from the same disease as persons. The virus that caused the 1918–1919 pandemic has been shown to be antigenically identical with porcine influenza virus (swine-flu virus). The virus was not studied during the pandemic itself; the methods for doing so were not developed until fifteen years later. In 1935, however, Andrewes showed that persons twenty years old or older had a high concentration of antibodies against swine-flu virus in their blood, whereas children younger than twelve had none. The clear conclusion is that swine-flu virus was infecting children at some time between 1915 and 1923, presumably 1918–1919.

Thorough studies have led to the classification of influenza viruses into several types, each with many strains. The types are A (with subtypes A_0, A_1, and A_2), B, and C. All non-human flu viruses are of type A. A person who has recovered from an infection with one type of the virus is immune to it for some time, but not to the others.

VACCINATION AGAINST INFLUENZA

Some protection against influenza is provided by the injection of a vaccine. The vaccine is prepared by growing the virus on embryonated (fertile) eggs, removing the allantoic fluid, which contains the crop of virus particles, and inactivating them by treatment with formaldehyde. The inactivated virus is no longer infective; that is, it is no longer able to stimulate the cells of a human being or other host to produce additional virus particles. It is, however, able to act as an antigen, causing the host to produce molecules of its specific antibody. This antibody can combine with active virus particles and neutralize them, thus protecting the immunized person against the disease.

Vaccines are usually made with strains of viruses that are prevalent in the country. Immunity from the vaccination lasts for about one year, after which booster doses extending the protection for another year may be given. The protection provided by vaccination is estimated to be 70 to 80 percent. Its failure may usually be ascribed to infection by a strain of virus differing from the strains used in making the vaccine; new strains seem to be continually arising. The partial protection provided by vaccination is considered to be especially important for old people and people with chronic diseases.

There are some possible side effects of the vaccination. Persons with a history of sensitivity to eggs should not be given the vaccine. Some persons suffer from local or systemic reactions to the vaccine, but immediate reactions followed by death are very rare. Because of the possible side effects, physicians usually advise their patients to be vaccinated only when there is a special reason. The imminence of an epidemic may constitute such a reason, especially for persons who, because of age or illness, are deficient in their natural protective mechanisms and for persons who are occupationally exposed, such as those in hospitals and clinics.

The importance of influenza is made clear by a 1973 report by Schmeck, based on unpublished data from the National Center for Health Statistics. In the ranking of diseases according to health impact in 1971, influenza and pneumonia (which often is a sequel to influenza) came first in days of disability in bed in 1971 (206,241,000), with upper respiratory infections second (164,840,000) and heart disease third (93,137,000). In deaths influenza and pneumonia rank fourth (56,000), behind heart disease (741,000), cancer (333,000), and cerebrovascular disease (208,000).

The best protection against the flu is one's natural defense mechanisms. These defense mechanisms seem to have protected about one-sixth of the people during the 1918–1919 pandemic, presumably for the most part those people whose defense mechanisms were operating most effectively. There is much evidence, some of which is discussed in later chapters, that a good intake of vitamin C improves the functioning of the natural defense mechanisms to such an extent that a much larger fraction of the population would resist the infection. The proper use of vitamin C, together with vaccination when its use is indicated, should be effective in preventing an influenza pandemic or serious epidemic.

3

Scurvy

Scurvy is a deficiency disease. It is caused by a deficiency of a certain food, vitamin C, in the diet. People who receive no vitamin C become sick and die.

Scurvy has been known for hundreds of years, but it was not until 1911 that its cause was clearly recognized to be a dietary deficiency. Until about a century ago the disease was very common among sailors on board ships taking long voyages. It also frequently broke out among soldiers in an army on campaign, in communities in times of scarcity of food, in cities under siege, and in prisons and workhouses. Scurvy plagued the California gold miners 130 years ago, and the Alaskan gold miners 80 years ago.

The onset of scurvy is marked by a failure of strength, including restlessness and rapid exhaustion on making effort. The skin becomes sallow or dusky. The patient complains of pains in the muscles. He is mentally depressed. Later, his face looks haggard. His gums ulcerate, his teeth drop out, and his breath is fetid. Hemorrhages of large size penetrate the muscles and other tissues, giving him the appearance of being extensively bruised. The later stages of the disease are marked by profound exhaustion, diarrhea, and pulmonary and kidney troubles, leading to death.

The ravages of scurvy among the early sea voyagers were terrible. On a long voyage the sailors lived largely on biscuits, salt beef, and salt pork, which contain very little vitamin C. Between 9 July 1497 and 20 May 1498 the Portuguese navigator Vasco da Gama made the voyage of discovery of the searoute around Africa to India, sailing from Lisbon to Calicut. During this voyage one hundred of his crew of 160 died of scurvy. In the year 1577 a Spanish galleon was found adrift in the Sargasso Sea, with everyone on board dead of scurvy. Late in 1740 the British Admiral George Anson set out with a squadron of six ships manned by 961 sailors. By June 1741, when he reached the island of Juan Fernandez, the number of sailors had decreased to 335, more than half of his men having died of scurvy.

The idea that scurvy could be prevented by a proper diet developed only slowly. In 1536 the French explorer Jacques Cartier discovered the St. Lawrence River, and sailed up the river to the site of the present city of Quebec, where Cartier and his men spent the winter. Twenty-five of the men died of scurvy, and many others were very sick. A friendly Indian advised them to make a tea with use of the leaves and bark of the arbor vitae tree, *Thuja occidentalis.* The treatment was beneficial. The leaves or needles of this tree have now been shown to contain about 50 mg of vitamin C per 100 g.

In 1747, while in the British naval service, the Scottish physician James Lind carried out a now famous experiment with twelve patients severely ill with scurvy. He placed them all on the same diet, except for one item, one or another of the reputed remedies that he was testing. To each of two patients he gave two oranges and one lemon per day; to two others, cider; to the others, dilute sulfuric acid, or vinegar, or sea water, or a mixture of drugs. At the end of six days the two who had received the citrus fruits were well, whereas the other ten remained ill. Lind carried out further studies, which he later described in his book, *A Treatise on Scurvy,* which was published in 1753.

There followed a period of controversy about the value of the juice of citrus fruits in preventing scurvy. Some of the unsuccessful trials involved the use of orange, lemon, and lime juice that had been boiled down to a syrup. We know now that most of the ascorbic acid in the juice was destroyed by this process. Finally, however, in 1795, forty-eight years after Lind had carried out his striking experiment, the British Admiralty ordered that a daily ration of lime juice* (not boiled to a syrup) be given to the sailors, and scurvy disappeared from the British Navy.

The spirit of free enterprise remained dominant in the British Board of Trade, however, and scurvy continued to ravage the British merchant marine for seventy years longer. In 1865 the Board of Trade finally passed a similar lime-juice regulation for the merchant marine.

The striking story of the experience of the great English explorer Captain James Cook in the control of scurvy among

---

*Hence the name Lime-juicer or Limey for an English sailor.

his crews on his Pacific voyages during the period 1768 to 1780 has been told by Kodicek and Young in the *Notes and Records of the Royal Society of London* (1969). These authors quote the following song by the sailor T. Perry, a member of the crew of Captain Cook's flagship H. M. S. Resolution:

> We were all hearty seamen, no colds did we fear
> And we have from all sickness entirely kept clear
> Thanks be to the Captain, he has proved so good
> Amongst all the Islands to give us fresh food.

This song, written two hundred years ago, indicates that Cook's sailors believed that fresh food (containing vitamin C) provided them with protection against colds, as well as against other diseases.

Captain Cook made use of many antiscorbutic agents. Whenever the ships reached shore he ordered the sailors to gather fruits, vegetables, berries, and green plants. In South America, Australia, and Alaska the leaves of spruce trees were gathered and made into an infusion called spruce beer. Nettletops and wild leeks were boiled with wheat and served at breakfast. Cook began one voyage with a supply of 7,860 pounds of sauerkraut, enough to provide two pounds per week for a period of a year for each of the seventy men on board his first flagship, the Endeavour. (Sauerkraut contains a good amount of vitamin C, about 30 mg per 100 g.) The result of his care was that, despite some illness, not a single member of his crew died of scurvy during his three Pacific voyages, carried out at a time when scurvy was still ravaging the crews of most vessels on such protracted voyages.

Cook was the son of a day laborer on a farm in Yorkshire. As a boy he showed unusual ability, and at age eighteen he was apprenticed to a ship owner, who encouraged him in his study of mathematics and navigation. After he joined the navy he advanced rapidly, and he became one of the world's greatest explorers. His scientific contributions were recognized by his election as a Fellow of the Royal Society of London, which awarded him the Copley Medal for his work on the prevention of scurvy.

The English admiral Sir John Hawkins (1532–1595) knew that the juice of citrus fruits is effective in preventing scurvy:

> It was found on a very long voyage that the crew suffered from scurvy in proportion to the length of time they were restricted to dry foods, and that they recovered rapidly as soon as they got access to a supply of succulent plants. This requisite for health is obviously the most difficult of all things to procure aboard ship, and efforts were made to find a substitute capable of marine transport. From the time of Hawkins (1593) downwards the opinion has been expressed by all the most intelligent travelers that a substitute is to be found in the juice of fruits of the orange tribes, such as oranges, lemons, etc. But in its natural state this is expensive and troublesome to carry, so that skippers and owners for a couple of centuries found it expedient to be skeptical. The pictures of scurvy as it appeared during the 18th century are horrible in the extreme. (In the article "Dietetics," *Encyclopedia Britannica*, 9th Edition, Volume 7, 1878.)

At the present time scurvy, complicated by other deficiency diseases, is found in populations that are ravaged by starvation and severe malnutrition, usually as a result of poverty. In the United States scurvy is also occasionally observed in people who are not poverty-stricken: among infants six to eighteen months old who are fed a formula without vitamin supplement, and such persons as middle-aged or elderly bachelors or widowers who for convenience ingest an unsatisfactory diet, deficient in the essential nutrients.

4

The Discovery
Of Vitamins

In the article on scurvy in the Eleventh Edition of the Encyclopedia Britannica (1911) the statement is made that the incidence of scurvy depends upon the nature of the food, and that it is disputed whether the cause is the *absence* of certain constituents in the food, or the *presence* of some actual poison.

The study of another disease, beriberi, was then in a similar state. Beriberi was prevalent in eastern Asia, where rice is the staple food, and was found also in the Pacific islands and South America. The disease involves paralysis and numbness, starting from the legs and leading to cardiac and respiratory disorders and to death. In the Dutch East Indies, about one hundred years ago, soldiers, sailors, prisoners, mine workers and plantation workers, and persons admitted to a hospital for treatment of minor ailments were dying of the disease by the thousands. Young men in seemingly good health sometimes died suddenly, in terrible distress through inability to breathe.

In 1886 a young Dutch physician, Christiaan Eijkman, was asked by the Dutch government to study the disease. For three years he made little progress. Then he noticed that the chickens in the laboratory chickenhouse were dying of a paralytic disease closely resembling beriberi. His studies of the chickens' disease were suddenly brought to an end, when the chickens that had not yet died recovered and no new cases developed. He found on investigating the circumstances that the man in charge of the chickens had been feeding them, from 17 June to 27 November, on polished rice (with the husks removed) prepared in the military hospital kitchen for the hospital patients. Then a new cook took charge of the kitchen; he refused to "allow military rice to be taken for civilian chickens."* The disease had broken out among the chickens on 10 July and disappeared during the last days of November.

It was immediately confirmed that a diet of polished rice causes death of chickens in three or four weeks, whereas they remain in good health when fed unpolished rice. A study of 300,000 prisoners in 101 prisons in the Dutch East Indies was then made, and it was found that the incidence of beriberi was three hundred times as great in the prisons where polished rice was used as a staple diet as in those where unpolished rice was used.

Eijkman found that he could isolate an extract from the bran of the rice that had protective power against beriberi. At first he thought that some substance in the bran acted as an antidote for a toxin assumed to be present in polished rice, but

---

*These are the words used by Eijkman in his Nobel address, when he received half of the Nobel Prize for Physiology and Medicine, 1929, awarded to him for his discovery of vitamin B_1, deficiency of which is the cause of beriberi.

by 1907 he and his collaborator Grijns had concluded that the bran contains a nutrient substance that is required for good health.

In the meantime a number of investigators had been studying the nutritional value of foods. It was shown that for good health certain minerals are needed (compounds of sodium, potassium, iron, copper, and other metals), as well as proteins, carbohydrates, and fats. The Swiss biochemist Lunin found, in 1881, that mice died when they were fed a mixture of purified protein, carbohydrate, fat, and minerals, whereas those fed the same diet with the addition of some milk survived. He concluded that "a natural food such as milk must therefore contain besides these known principal ingredients small quantities of unknown substances essential to life." Similar observations were made in the same laboratory (in Basel) ten years later by another Swiss biochemist, Socin, who found that small amounts of either egg yolk or milk, in addition to the purified diet, sufficed to keep the mice in good health. In 1905 the Dutch physiologist Pekelharing found that very small amounts of the unknown essential substances in milk were enough to keep the animals in good health. Between 1905 and 1912 the English biochemist F. Gowland Hopkins carried on similar studies with rats, showing that, in addition to purified protein, carbohydrate, fat, and minerals, a small amount of milk is needed to keep the rats in good health. His results were announced in 1911 and published in detail in 1912. Hopkins shared the 1929 Nobel Prize for Physiology and Medicine with Eijkman.

In 1911 Casimir Funk, a Polish biochemist then working in the Lister Institute in London, published his theory of "vitamines," based upon his review of the existing knowledge about diseases associated with faulty nutrition. He suggested that four such substances are present in natural foods, and that they serve to provide protection against four diseases, beriberi, scurvy, pellagra, and rickets. Funk coined the word vitamine from the Latin word *vita,* life, and the chemical term amine, a member of a class of compounds of nitrogen. Later, when it was found that some of these essential substances do not contain nitrogen, the word was changed to vitamin.

During the following years a number of efforts were made to isolate pure vitamin C from lemon juice and other foods. The pure vitamin was finally obtained, in 1928, by a scientist, Albert Szent-Györgyi, who was working on another problem, and at first did not know that his new substance was vitamin C. He named the substance hexuronic acid, and later changed the name to ascorbic acid. Szent-Györgyi was given the Nobel Prize for Physiology and Medicine for the year 1937, in recognition of his discoveries concerning the biological oxidation processes, with especial reference to vitamin C and to the role of fumaric acid in these processes.

Albert Szent-Györgyi was born in Budapest on 16 September 1893. He studied medicine in Budapest, and immediately began his career as an investigator in the fields of physiology and biochemistry. While he was working in the Netherlands in 1922 he began a study of the oxidation reactions that cause a brown pigmentation to appear in certain fruits, such as apples and bananas, as they decay. In the course of these studies he found that cabbages contain a reducing agent (an agent that can combine with oxygen), and that the adrenal glands of animals contain the same reducing agent, or a similar one. Because of his interest in physiological oxidation-reduction reactions he began to try to isolate this reducing agent from the plant tissues and from adrenal glands.

In 1927 he received a fellowship from the Rockefeller Foundation, permitting him to spend a year in the laboratory of F. Gowland Hopkins in Cambridge, England. Here he succeeded in isolating the substance from plant tissues and from the adrenal glands of animals. He then spent a year in the Mayo Foundation, Rochester, Minnesota, where he succeeded in obtaining 25 grams of the substance, which he called hexuronic acid. In 1930 he returned to Hungary, where he found that Hungarian paprika contains large amounts of the substance. He and his collaborators, and also the American investigators Waugh and King, showed in 1932 that Szent-Györgyi's substance was vitamin C. Szent-Györgyi himself had found that the chemical formula of the substance is $C_6H_8O_6$. He gave some of the crystalline material to the English sugar chemist W. M. Haworth, who determined its structural formula. Szent-Györgyi and Haworth then changed its name to ascorbic acid, meaning the acidic substance that prevents scurvy.

Within a short time the value of ascorbic acid in improving health began to be recognized. The pure substance soon became available in drug stores and food stores. For many years, however, there was an astounding lack of interest by physicians in the use of this important food for the benefit of their patients. At the present time, however, the attitude of physicians toward ascorbic acid and other important nutrients is undergoing a significant change, in part because of new evidence that has been gathered, some of which is described in the following chapters of this book. It is also being increasingly recognized that the intake of other vitamins and of some nonessential nutritional factors can be varied in such a way as to produce a significant improvement in general health and a decrease in the incidence and severity of disease.

5

Ascorbic Acid

Ascorbic acid is an essential food for human beings. As noted earlier, an intake of about 10 mg per day is enough to provide protection against scurvy for most people, but to achieve the best health a much larger intake is probably needed.

The optimum intake of ascorbic acid — that is, the daily amount of this food that leads to the best of health — is not known with certainty, and no doubt it varies from person to person. It is my opinion that for most people the optimum daily intake is somewhere between 250 mg and 10 g.

These amounts are much larger than the daily dietary allowance recommended in 1974 by the Food and Nutrition Board of the National Research Council. The recommendation of this Board, said to be designed for the maintenance of good nutrition of practically all healthy people in the United States, is 35 mg per day for infants, 40 mg per day for children, increasing to 45 mg per day for adults (60 for pregnant women and 80 for lactating women). In making its recommendation the Board stated that the minimum daily intake of ascorbic acid needed to prevent scurvy is about 10 mg, and that the somewhat larger amounts recommended should provide a generous increment for individual variability and a surplus to compensate for potential losses in food. The idea that beneficial effects would result from a larger intake of ascorbic acid was rejected, on the basis of reports that improvement in physical and psychomotor performances of men had not been improved by supplements of between 70 mg and 300 mg of ascorbic acid per day, and that the occurrence of bleeding gums in military personnel was not affected by supplements of 100 mg or 200 mg per day for periods of three weeks. There are, however, many published reports about beneficial effects of ascorbic acid ingested in larger amounts. Some of these reports are discussed later in this chapter and in the following chapters and Appendix III.

Ascorbic acid is not a dangerous substance. It is described in the medical literature as "virtually nontoxic." Guinea pigs that were given, orally or by intravenous infusion (of sodium ascorbate, the sodium salt of ascorbic acid), one half of one percent of their body weight per day for a period of days showed no symptoms of toxicity (Demole, 1934). This amount corresponds for a human being to about 350 g (three quarters of a pound) per day. Many dogs and cats have been given large doses for control of distemper, influenza, rhinotracheitis, cystitis, and other diseases, with beneficial results and no signs of toxicity (Belfield and Stone, 1975). The amount used was 1 g per pound of body weight per day, injected intravenously (in two doses, morning and afternoon), corresponding to about 150 g per day for an adult human being. Human beings themselves have taken 10 to 20 g of vitamin C every day for 25 years with no development of kidney stones or other side effects (Klenner, 1971; Stone, 1967). Patients with glaucoma have been treated with about 35 g of vitamin C (0.5 g per kilogram body weight) each day for more than seven months (Virno et al., 1967; Bietti, 1967). The only side effect reported was diarrhea during the first three to four days. Patients with viral diseases or schizophrenia have received as much as 100 g per day with no symptoms of toxicity (Klenner, 1971; Herjanic and Moss-Herjanic, 1967). A large amount (several grams) of ascorbic acid taken without other food may cause an upset stomach and diarrhea in some people (hence the recommendation in Chapter 14 that it usually be taken at the end of a meal), but more serious side effects have not been reported.

A thorough discussion of possible side effects of large doses of ascorbic acid is given in Chapter 11.

Ascorbic acid may be described as no more toxic than ordinary sugar (sucrose), and far less toxic than ordinary salt (sodium chloride). There is no reported case of the death of any person from eating too much ascorbic acid, nor, indeed, of serious illness from this cause.

Ascorbic acid is a white, crystalline powder, with large solubility in water. Its solution has an acidic taste, resembling that of orange juice.

Ordinary ascorbic acid is also called L-ascorbic acid. There is another substance, D-ascorbic acid, that is closely related to L-ascorbic acid; the two substances contain the same atoms, bonded together in essentially the same way, but with a spatial relationship corresponding to reflection in a mirror. The letters D and L indicate righthanded (dextro) and lefthanded (levo). Only L-ascorbic acid has vitamin-C activity. The name ascorbic acid without a prefix is used only in refering to L-ascorbic acid, vitamin C itself.

Ascorbic acid is found in many foodstuffs. Large amounts, 100 mg to 350 mg per 100 g (that is, between 0.10 and 0.35 percent of the weight of the food) are contained in green peppers, red peppers, parsley, and turnip greens. Orange juice, lemon juice, lime juice, grapefruit juice, tomato juice, mustard greens, spinach, and brussels sprouts contain a good quantity of ascorbic acid, from 25 mg to 100 mg per 100 g. Green peas and green beans, sweet corn, asparagus, pineapple, tomatoes, gooseberries, cranberries, cucumbers, and lettuce contain from 10 mg to 25 mg per 100 g. Somewhat smaller amounts—less than 10 mg per 100 g—are found in eggs, milk, carrots, beets, and cooked meat.

The ascorbic acid in foodstuffs is easily destroyed by cooking at high temperatures, especially in the presence of copper and to some extent of other metals. Cooked foods usually retain only about half of the ascorbic acid present in the raw foods. The loss of the vitamin can be kept to a minimum by cooking for a short period of time, with a minimum amount of water and with the water not discarded, because it has extracted some of the vitamin from the food.

A good ordinary diet, including green vegetables and orange or tomato juice, may provide 100 mg of ascorbic acid per day. Many people, however, do not obtain even this rather small amount. In the 1971–1972 study by the Health Resources Administration of the U.S. Department of Health, Education, and Welfare of 10,126 people of age one to seventy-four years in ten representative geographical areas of the country, it was found that half of the people receive less than 57.9 mg of vitamin C per day and about one-third of the people receive less than the RDA (recommended dietary allowance), which is

45 mg per day for an adult (Abraham et al., 1976). Only 30 percent have a daily intake greater than 100 mg, and only 17 percent greater than 150 mg. The average intake of people below the poverty level is 78 percent that of the whole population, and 57 percent of them receive less than the RDA.

To obtain larger amounts of this important food, the pure substance, crystalline ascorbic acid, may be ingested.

Pure ascorbic acid (Ascorbic Acid U.S.P., L-Ascorbic Acid, Vitamin C) is available in some drug stores and food stores as a powder, fine crystals, or coarse crystals, and also, with a binder or filler added, as tablets. This ascorbic acid is sometimes described as synthetic ascorbic acid. It is identical with the ascorbic acid present in natural foodstuffs, and it is, in fact, usually made from a natural sugar by a process involving two chemical reactions. The usual starting material is dextrose, which is also called glucose, grape sugar, honey sugar, corn sugar, or starch sugar. It is present in honey and other natural foods. Its chemical formula is $C_6H_{12}O_6$. It is converted into L-ascorbic acid, $C_6H_8O_6$, by oxidation reactions which remove four hydrogen atoms to form two molecules of water.

Many animals are able to manufacture their own ascorbic acid; they do not require ascorbic acid (vitamin C) as an essential food, and they never suffer from scurvy. These animals manufacture the ascorbic acid in their bodies (in the liver or the kidney) from dextrose by essentially the same reactions that are used to make ascorbic acid in the laboratory and on a commercial scale.

Ascorbic acid in the human body and in other animals seems to have many functions. These functions have been studied in the guinea pig and the monkey, both of which, like human beings, require ascorbic acid in their food, as a vitamin. It has been found that an insufficient supply of this essential food causes the animal to show symptoms of scurvy, including intramuscular and subcutaneous hemorrhages, tenderness of joints, a general weakening of connective tissue (skin, tendons, walls of blood vessels), lethargy, loss of appetite, and anemia. Ascorbic acid is needed for the healing of wounds, including burns. With a low intake of ascorbic acid wounds heal only slowly and the scar tissue is weak, so that the wounds break open again easily. Increase in the intake of ascorbic acid leads to rapid healing and to the formation of strong scar tissue (see Figure 1).

It has been found that a large intake of ascorbic acid increases the capacity of resistance of the guinea pig, the rat, and the monkey to a cold environment (Dugal, 1961). In human beings, a fall in the concentration of ascorbic acid in the blood has been observed to follow exposure to the stress of surgery, accidental wounds, and burns, indicating the need for a larger supply of the vitamin. Ascorbic acid in increased amounts has been used in the treatment of burns, injuries, infections, rheumatic disease, and allergies (Holmes, 1946; Yandell, 1951).

In 1964 Dr. James Greenwood, Jr., clinical professor of neurosurgery in Baylor University College of Medicine, reported his observations on the effect of an increased intake of ascorbic acid in preserving the integrity of intervertebral discs and preventing back trouble. He recommended the use of 500 mg per day with an increase to 1,000 mg per day if there were any discomfort or if work or strenuous exercise were anticipated. He said that evidence from most patients indicated that muscular soreness experienced with exercise had been greatly reduced by these doses of ascorbic acid, but increased again when the vitamin was not taken. He concluded, from observation of over 500 cases, that "it can be stated with

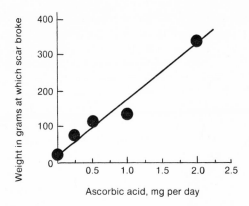

FIGURE 1
Strength of scar tissue in guinea-pig skin in dependence on the amount of ascorbic acid in the diet (0, 0.25, 0.5, 1, and 2 mg per day). The scars had been formed during a seven-day period after the cuts, ¼-inch long, had been made. It is seen that the scar tissue is four times as strong for an intake of 2 mg per day as for 0.25 mg per day (Bourne, 1946). Similar results for human beings have been reported by Wolfer, Farmer, Carroll, and Manshardt (1947)

reasonable assurance that a significant percentage of patients with early disc lesions were able to avoid surgery by the use of large doses of vitamin C. Many of these patients after a few months or years stopped their vitamin C and symptoms recurred. When they were placed back on the vitamin the symptoms disappeared. Some, of course, eventually came to surgery."

It has also been reported that the cancers that often appear in the bladders of cigar smokers and other users of tobacco regress if the patient ingests a sufficient amount of ascorbic acid, 1 g per day or more. Schlegel, Pipkin, Nishimura, and Schultz (1970) found the ascorbic-acid level of the urine to be about half as great for smokers as for nonsmokers, and to be low for patients with bladder tumors. They also found with mice that implantation in the bladder of a pellet containing 3-hydroxyanthranilic acid (a derivative of the amino acid tryptophan) caused bladder tumors to develop if the mice were receiving a normal diet, but not if they had extra acorbic acid in their drinking water. The authors suggest that the ascorbic acid prevents the oxidation of 3-hydroxyanthranilic acid to a cancerogenic oxidation product. They state that "there seems to be reason to consider the beneficial effects of an adequate ascorbic acid level in the urine (corresponding to a rate of intake of 1.5 g per day) as a possible preventive measure in regard to bladder tumor formation and recurrence." They also call attention to investigations indicating that ascorbic acid may have a beneficial effect on the aging process of atherosclerosis, the hardening and thickening of the walls of the arteries (Willis and Fishman, 1955; Sokoloff and others, 1966).

Patients with various infectious diseases have been reported to benefit from treatment with ascorbic acid. Some of the reports are discussed in later chapters of this book.

An interesting investigation of the relation between intelligence, as indicated by the results of standard mental ability tests, and the concentration of ascorbic acid in the blood plasma has been reported by Kubala and Katz (1960). The subjects were 351 students in four schools (kindergarten to college) in three cities. They were initially divided into the higher-ascorbic-acid group (with more than 1.10 mg of ascorbic acid per 100 ml of blood plasma) and the lower-ascorbic-acid group (less than 1.10 mg per 100 ml) on the basis of analysis of blood samples. By matching pairs on a socio-economic basis (family income, education of father and mother), seventy-two subjects in the higher-ascorbic-acid group and seventy-two in the lower-ascorbic-acid group were selected. It was found that the average intelligence quotient of the higher-ascorbic-acid group was greater than that of the lower-ascorbic-acid group in each of the four schools; for all seventy-two pairs of subjects the average IQ values were 113.22 and 108.71, respectively, with an average difference 4.51. The probability that a difference this great would be found in a similar test on a uniform population is less than 5 percent: hence the observed difference in average IQ of the two groups is statistically significant.

The subjects in both groups were then given supplementary orange juice during a period of six months, and the tests were repeated. The average intelligence quotient for those in the initially higher-ascorbic-acid group had increased very little (by only 0.02), whereas that for the lower group had increased by 3.54 IQ units. This difference in increase is also statistically significant (with a probability of less than 5 percent in a uniform population).

The study was continued through a second school year with thirty-two pairs (sixty-four subjects), with similar results. The relation between the average intelligence quotient and the average blood-plasma ascorbic-acid concentration for these sixty-four subjects tested four times during a period of months is shown in Figure 2. These results indicate that the intelligence quotient is raised by 3.6 IQ units when the blood-plasma ascorbic-acid concentration is increased by 50 percent (from 1.03 to 1.55 mg per 100 ml). This increase would for many people result from increasing the intake of ascorbic acid for an adult by 50 mg per day (from 100 mg to 150 mg per day).

Kubala and Katz conclude that some of the variance in intelligence-test performance is determined by the "temporary nutritional state of the individual, at least with regards to citrus or other products providing ascorbic acid." They suggest that "alertness" or "sharpness" is diminished by a decreased intake of ascorbic acid.

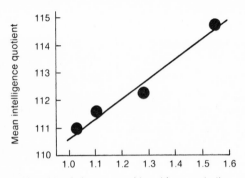

FIGURE 2

Relation between mean intelligence quotient (average IQ) and mean concentration of ascorbic acid in the blood plasma for sixty-four school children. Four tests were made of each child, over a period of eighteen months. The plasma ascorbic-acid concentration was changed by giving all the subjects extra orange juice during certain months. (Redrawn from Figure 1 of Kubala and Katz, 1960).

There is no indication in Figure 2 that maximum mental ability has been reached at the value 1.55 mg of ascorbic acid per 100 ml of blood plasma. This concentration corresponds for a 70-kg (154-pound) adult to the daily ingestion of about 180 mg of ascorbic acid. I conclude that for maximum mental performance the daily allowance of ascorbic acid should be at least four times the 45 mg recommended by the Food and

Nutrition Board of the U.S. National Research Council, and at least nine times the 20 mg recommended by the corresponding British authority.

The ways in which ascorbic acid functions in the human body are only partially understood. It is a strong reducing agent, and is readily converted into dehydroascorbic acid, $C_6H_6O_6$, by oxidizing agents:

Ascorbic acid   Dehydroascorbic acid

This reaction is reversible (dehydroascorbic acid is easily reduced to ascorbic acid), and it is likely that the reducing power of ascorbic acid and the oxidizing power of dehydro-ascorbic acid are responsible for some of the physiological properties of the substance.

Many of the results of deprivation of ascorbic acid, mentioned above, involve a deficiency in connective tissue. Connective tissue is largely responsible for the strength of bones, teeth, skin, tendons, blood-vessel walls, and other parts of the body. It consists mainly of the fibrous protein collagen. There is no doubt that ascorbic acid is required for the synthesis of collagen in the bodies of human beings and other animals.

Collagen differs from other fibrous proteins in having a rather large content of the amino acid hydroxyproline. There is evidence that ascorbic acid is required for the conversion of prolyl residues of procollagen, the precursor of collagen, into the hydroxyprolyl residues that give collagen its characteristic properties, making it a valuable constituent of the tissues of the human body. This is an oxidation reaction, and there is evidence also that ascorbic acid is involved in some other oxidation reactions in the tissues.

One of the important functions of collagen is its service in strengthening the intercellular cement that holds the cells of the body together in various tissues. The intercellular cement contains a mucopolysaccharide, called hyaluronic acid, in which tiny fibrils of collagen are embedded. These fibrils are not synthesized when the intake of vitamin C is low. In his book *The Advancing Front of Medicine* (1941) an able science writer, George W. Gray, who was associated with the Rockefeller Foundation, wrote the following statement about ascorbic acid:

> Recent studies show that vitamin C is essential to the formation of the colloidal substance which serves as a pliable cement to bind tissue cells together. In healthy tissue, this binding material shows under the microscope as a clear jelly streaked with darker bands of firmer texture, like the reinforcing strips of steel in concrete. But in the absence of sufficient vitamin C, the bands do not form, the intercellular substance becomes more liquid, less binding, and the cells show a tendency to separate. The hemorrhages which accompany scurvy are consequences of this weakness in the intercellular substance. The cells forming the walls of small blood vessels separate, and through the gaps the blood leaks out. Microscopic studies show that as soon as vitamin C is administered to a scurvy patient, the bands

reappear in the intercellular substance, and the separated cells once more join into continuous tissue.

It is not unlikely that part of the effectiveness of vitamin C against the common cold, influenza, and other viral diseases can be attributed to its action in strengthening the intercellular cement and in this way preventing or hindering the motion of the virus particles through the tissues and into the cells (Pauling, 1973a).

Ascorbic acid is a weak acid, somewhat stronger than acetic acid, found in vinegar, but weaker than citric acid (lemons and grapefruit), lactic acid (sour milk and sauerkraut), and tartaric acid (grapes). In body fluids, which are usually neither acidic nor basic, ascorbic acid is completely dissociated into hydrogen ion, which combines with basic groups of proteins or with carbonate ion. The ascorbate ion gives to vitamin C its power to prevent scurvy by permitting collagen to be synthesized and by participating in other physiological reactions. The salts of ascorbic acid, in particular sodium ascorbate and calcium ascorbate, also dissociate to produce ascorbate ion, which has the same properties as ascorbate ion from ascorbic acid. Vitamin C may be taken by mouth as ascorbic acid, sodium ascorbate, or calcium ascorbate, but only the salts can be injected, because the acid damages the veins or tissues.

In 1970, I formulated the hypothesis that vitamin C also is involved in the synthesis and activity of interferon in preventing the entry of virus particles into the cells. The discovery of interferon was reported in 1957 by Isaacs and Lindenmann. Interferon is a protein that is produced by cells infected by a virus and that has the property of spreading to neighboring cells and changing them in such a way as to enable them to resist infection. In this way the interferon ameliorates the disease. There was no direct evidence about the interaction of vitamin C and interferon in 1970, but some has been reported recently (Schwerdt and Schwerdt, 1975).

6

Ascorbic Acid and the Common Cold

I mentioned in the Introduction my decision to try to resolve the apparent contradiction between the opinions expressed by authorities in nutrition and my own experience, which supported the widely held belief that ascorbic acid has value in decreasing the incidence of infection and ameliorating the severity of the common cold.

The solution to the puzzle is a simple one. Ascorbic acid has only rather small value in providing protection against the common cold when it is taken in small amounts, but it has great value when it is taken in large amounts. As is explained below, the amount of protection increases with increase in the amount of ingested ascorbic acid, and becomes nearly complete with 4 g to 10 g per day taken at the immediate onset of the cold, as recommended by Irwin Stone and Edmé Régnier.

Most of the studies referred to in the editorial article in the August 1967 issue of *Nutrition Reviews* involved giving small amounts of ascorbic acid to the subjects, usually 200 mg per day. These studies indicate that such small amounts of ascorbic acid have some protective value, not very great, against the common cold.

The study of vitamin C in relation to the common cold began only a few years after the vitamin was identified as ascorbic acid. In 1938 Dr. Roger Korbsch of St. Elisabeth Hospital, Oberhausen, Germany, published an account of his observations. The fact that ascorbic acid had been reported to be effective against several diseases, including gastritis and stomach ulcers, suggested that he try it in treating acute rhinitis and colds. In 1936 he found that oral doses of up to 1 g per day were of value against rhinorrhea, acute rhinitis, and secondary rhinitis and accompanying manifestations of illness, such as headache. He then found that the injection of 250 or 500 mg of ascorbic acid on the first day of a common cold almost always led to the immediate disappearance of all the signs and symptoms of the cold, with a similar injection sometimes needed on the second day. He stated that ascorbic acid is far superior to other cold medicines, such as aminopyrine, and is without danger, in that there is no evidence that there are serious side effects, even with large doses.

A trial was then made in Germany (Ertel, 1941) in which 357 million daily doses of vitamin C were distributed among 3.7 million pregnant women, nursing mothers, suckling infants, and school children. Ertel reported that the recipients of the vitamin C enjoyed better health, in several different respects, than the corresponding control populations. The only quantitative information given by him is that with one group of school children for which good statistical data were collected the amount of illness with respiratory infections was 20 percent less than the year before.

In 1942 Glazebrook and Thomson reported the results of a study carried out in an institution where there were about 1,500 students, whose ages ranged from fifteen to twenty years. The food was poorly prepared, being kept hot for two hours or more before serving, and the total intake of ascorbic acid was determined to be only about 5 mg to 15 mg per student per day. Some of the students (335) were given additional ascorbic acid, 200 mg per day, for a period of six months, and the others (1,100) were kept as controls. The incidence of colds and tonsillitis was 30.1 percent in the ascorbic-acid group during this period, and that in the controls was 34.5 percent. Thus there were 13 percent fewer colds among the students given ascorbic acid than among the controls. Students with moderately severe colds or tonsillitis were admitted to the Sick Quarters of the institution. Of the students receiving ascorbic acid 23.0 percent were admitted to Sick Quarters, as compared with 30.5 percent of the controls. Accordingly the number of serious cases of colds or tonsillitis, requiring admission to Sick Quarters, was 25 percent less for the students receiving ascorbic acid than for the controls. This difference has high statistical significance (only 1 percent probability in a uniform population).

The average number of days of hospitalization per student because of infection (common cold, tonsillitis, acute rheumatism, pneumonia) was 2.5 for the students receiving ascorbic acid and 5.0 days for the controls. There were seventeen cases of pneumonia and sixteen cases of acute rheumatism among the 1,100 controls, and no case of either disease among the 335 students receiving ascorbic acid. The probability of such a great difference in two samples of a uniform population is so small (less than 0.3 percent) as to indicate very strongly that ascorbic acid has value in providing protection against these serious infectious diseases, as well as against the common cold and tonsillitis.

In carrying out such a test, the best experiments are those in which the subjects are divided into two groups, in a random way, with the substance being tested (ascorbic acid) administered to the subjects in one group, and a placebo (an inactive material resembling the preparation to be tested: for example, a capsule containing citric acid might be used as a placebo for ascorbic acid) administered to those of the other group. In a blind experiment the subjects do not know whether or not they are receiving the placebo. Sometimes a double-blind study is made, in which the investigators evaluating the effects of the preparation and the placebo do not know which of the subjects received the preparation and which received the placebo until the study is completed, this information being kept by some other person.

In 1942 Cowan, Diehl, and Baker published an account in the *Journal of the American Medical Association* of a study that they had made of the incidence of colds in students in the University of Minnesota during the winter of 1939–1940.* The students had volunteered to participate in the study because they were particularly susceptible to colds. About four hun-

---

*This is the study mentioned, rather inaccurately, by Dr. Fredrick J. Stare, who was quoted in the 1969 *Mademoiselle* article, and described by him as "a very careful study" (see the Introduction).

dred students participated in the study. About half of them received vitamin C, usually two 100-mg tablets per day, for a total of twenty-eight weeks, and the other half received a placebo. These students did not know that they were serving as controls.*

The investigators concluded that this amount of ascorbic acid, about 200 mg per day, did not have an important effect on the number or severity of infections of the upper respiratory tract when administered to young adults who presumably were already on a reasonably adequate diet. They obtained, however, three results that have significance. First, the average number of colds per person receiving ascorbic acid during the period of twenty-eight weeks was 1.9 ± 0.07, whereas the average number of colds in the control group was 2.2 ± 0.08 (Cowan, Diehl, and Baker should have reported their results to one more significant figure). The investigators conclude that "the actual difference between the two groups during the year of the study amounts to $\frac{1}{3}$ of a cold per person. Statistical analysis of the data reveals that a difference as large as this would arise only three or four times in a hundred through

---

*The Editor of the *Journal of the American Medical Association* asked me if the study by Cowan, Diehl, and Baker was a double-blind one. The answer is given in the following sentences from the letter of 2 February 1971 from Dr. Donald W. Cowan to me: "I have your letters of January 25 and 26, but unfortunately I am unable to answer your questions. We made quite a search of our dusty files in the basement but were unable to locate the original data upon which the report was based. This material no doubt was destroyed long since to make way for records more recently acquired. I can say that the study was double blind in nature, which answers one of your questions. . . . I have sent copies of your letters to Drs. Diehl and Baker, together with this reply, with the thought that they might wish to reply also." Neither Dr. Diehl nor Dr. Baker commented on the statement that the study was double blind in nature.

chance alone. One may therefore consider this as probably a significant difference, and vitamin C supplements to the diet may therefore be judged to give a slight advantage in reducing the number of colds experienced. However, one may well question the practical importance of such a difference."

This difference, one third, represents a decrease in the number of colds during the winter by 15 percent, 0.33/2.2, apparently resulting from ingestion of 200 mg of ascorbic acid per day. I think that such a difference does have practical importance. Also, the investigators might have asked whether taking twice as much ascorbic acid, 400 mg per day, would have decreased the number of colds by twice as much, 30 percent.

There is a second interesting aspect of the study made by Cowan, Diehl, and Baker. The ascorbic-acid group began with 233 students, of whom 25 dropped out during the twenty-eight weeks of the study. The control group began with 194 students, of whom 39 dropped out. Thus 20 percent of the control group dropped out of the study, and only 10 percent of those receiving ascorbic acid. The chance that this difference in the fraction of dropouts would occur in two samples of a uniform population is only 1 percent. Hence it seems likely that the population was not uniform in this respect; instead, a larger fraction of the students receiving ascorbic acid felt that they were benefited by the treatment than of those receiving the placebo.

A third aspect of the study is also statistically significant. The students who received the placebo lost an average of 1.6 days from school because of colds, and those who received ascorbic acid lost only an average of 1.1 days, 3 percent less. The probability that this difference would occur in a uniform population is only 0.1 percent, so that it is highly likely that the decrease in the amount of illness was caused by the ascorbic acid. A summary of the results reported by Cowan, Diehl, and Baker is given in Table 1.

TABLE 1
Results of the investigation by Cowan, Diehl, and Baker (1942)

	Placebo Group	Ascorbic-acid Group	Decrease
Number in group	155	208	
Incidence of (colds per person during the study)	2.2	1.9	15%
Severity (days of illness per cold)	0.73	0.58	21%
Integrated morbidity (days of illness per person)	1.6	1.1	31%

The results of the first carefully controlled study with a larger daily amount, 1,000 mg, of ascorbic acid were reported in 1961 by Dr. G. Ritzel, who is a physician with the medical service of the School District of the city of Basel, Switzerland. The study was carried out in a ski resort with 279 boys during two periods of five to seven days. The conditions were such that the incidence of colds during these short periods was large enough (approximately 20 percent) to permit results with statistical significance to be obtained. The subjects were of the same age (fifteen to seventeen) and had similar nutrition during the period of study. The investigation was double blind, with neither the participants nor the physicians having any knowledge about the distribution of the ascorbic-acid tablets (1,000 mg) and the placebo tablets. The tablets were distributed every morning and taken by the subjects under observation in such a way that the possibility of interchange of tablets was eliminated. The subjects were examined daily for symptoms of colds and other infections, as listed in the footnote to Table 2. The records were largely on the basis of subjective symptoms, partially supported by objective observations (measurement of body temperature, inspection of the respiratory organs, auscultation of the lungs, and so on). Persons who showed cold symptoms on the first day were excluded from the investigation.

After the completion of the investigation a completely independent group of professional people was provided with the identification numbers for the ascorbic acid tablets and

TABLE 2
Results of the investigation by Ritzel (1961)

	Placebo Group	Ascorbic-acid Group	Decrease
Number in group	140	139	
Number of colds	31	17	
Incidence of colds	0.221	0.122	45%
Total days of illness	80	31	
Total individual symptoms*	119	42	
Severity of individual colds, from days of illness per cold	2.58	1.82	29%
from individual symptoms per cold	3.84	2.47	36%
Integrated morbidity from days of illness per person	0.571	0.223	61%
from individual symptoms per person	0.850	0.302	64%

*Pharyngitis, laryngitis, tonsillitis, sore throat; bronchitis, coughing; fever, chills; otitis media; rhinitis; herpes labialis; other symptoms (muscle ache, headache, abdominal pain, vomiting, diarrhea, general malaise).

placebo tablets, and this group carried out the statistical evaluation of the observations.

The principal results of the investigation are given in Table 2. Ritzel pointed out that the group receiving ascorbic acid showed only 39 percent as many days of illness per person as the group receiving the placebo, that the number of individual symptoms per person was only 36 percent as great for the ascorbic-acid group as for the placebo group, and that the statistical evaluation showed that these differences are statistically significant at better than the 99-percent level of confidence. He also pointed out that the average number of days per cold for the ascorbic-acid group was 1.8 (more accurately 1.82), 29 percent less than the value for the placebo group, 2.6 (2.58), and that this difference is statistically significant.

In the paper by Ritzel the values of the number of patients showing different symptoms (the seven classes of symptoms listed in the footnote to Table 2) are given, and the number of days of illness for each symptom. It is interesting that for each of these seven classes of symptoms the number of patients showing the symptom is less for the ascorbic-acid group than for the placebo group, and that, moreover, the number of days of illness per patient showing the symptom is also less.

We see that in Ritzel's study the ascorbic-acid subjects had only about one-third as much illness as the placebo subjects.*

Since the publication of my book *Vitamin C and the Common Cold* in 1970, several excellent double-blind studies

---

*A serious error in reporting the results of this investigation was made by the author of the editorial article in *Nutrition Reviews* mentioned in the Introduction, where it is stated that there was only 39 percent reduction in the number of days of illness and 35 percent reduction in the incidence of symptoms. This error may have contributed to the unfavorable opinion expressed in the article.

have been carried out. The first one, in Toronto, Canada (Anderson, Reid, and Beaton, 1972), involved 407 subjects receiving ascorbic acid (1 g per day plus 3 g per day for three days at the onset of any illness) and 411 subjects receiving a closely matching placebo. The duration of the study was four months. The number of days confined to house per subject was 30 percent less for the ascorbic-acid group than for the placebo group, and the number of days off work per subject was 33 percent less. The authors mention that these differences have high statistical significance (99.9 percent level of confidence).

Another double-blind study (Coulehan, Resinger, Rogers, and Bradley, 1974) involved 641 children in a Navajo boarding school. The older children received 2 g of ascorbic acid per day (or a placebo), and the younger ones 1 g. During the study, which lasted fourteen weeks, the average number of days of illness with colds per child was 30 percent less for the 321 ascorbic-acid subjects than for the 320 placebo subjects, and the number of days with illness other than respiratory was 17 percent less. The differences have statistical significance. Another study, under quite different conditions, involved 112 soldiers undergoing operational training in northern Canada (Sabiston and Radomski, 1974). Half of the subjects received 1 g of ascorbic acid per day during the four weeks of the study, and the other half received a placebo. The average number of days of illness was 68 percent less for the ascorbic-acid subjects than for the placebo subjects.

The average amount of protection against the common cold found in these four studies in which 1 g or 2 g was given per day is 48 percent; that is, on the average the subjects who received the inactive tablet. This conclusion is supported also by the results of the other studies that have been made, as described in Appendix III.

Moreover, whether or not you take vitamin C regularly, almost every cold can be prevented or stopped by taking a large amount, several grams, when you think that you are in danger of catching a cold or that a cold is beginning. In 1938 Ruskin reported his observations on over one thousand patients whom he had given an injection, sometimes followed by a second one, of 450 mg of calcium ascorbate (the calcium salt of L-ascorbic acid) as soon as possible after the onset of a cold. He found that 42 percent of the patients were completely relieved and another 48 percent were markedly improved. He concluded that "calcium ascorbate would appear to be practically an abortive in the treatment of the common cold." Several other somewhat similar reports are mentioned by Stone in his book *The Healing Factor: Vitamin C Against Disease* (1972). Stone himself recommends taking 1.5 to 2 g of ascorbic acid by mouth at the first sign of a cold, with the dose repeated at twenty-minute to half-hour intervals until the symptoms have disappeared, which occurs usually by the third dose.

The physician Edmé Régnier of Salem, Massachusetts, reported in 1968 that he had discovered the value of the administration of large doses of ascorbic acid in the prevention and treatment of the common cold. For many years, beginning at the age of seven, he had suffered from repeated bouts of inflammation of the middle ear. He had tried a number of ways of controlling the infections, and after twenty years he made a trial of the bioflavonoids (vitamin P complex, from citrus fruits) and ascorbic acid. He felt that this treatment had been of some benefit, but not very great. He decided to try increasing the amount. After several trials he found that the serious and disagreeable manifestations of the common cold and the accompanying inflammation of the middle ear could be averted by the use of large amounts of ascorbic acid, and that ascorbic acid alone was just as effective as the same amount of ascorbic acid plus bioflavonoids. He initiated a study of twenty-two subjects with use of ascorbic acid alone, ascorbic acid plus bioflavonoids, bioflavonoids alone, or a placebo. This study extended over a period of five years. At first the subjects were kept ignorant of the preparations that they received, but later on (during the last year) it became impossible to continue the blind study, because a patient whose cold was developing recognized that he was not receiving the vitamin C that might have prevented it.

The method of treatment recommended by Dr. Régnier is the administration of 600 mg of ascorbic acid at the first signs of a cold (scratchiness of the throat, nasal secretion, sneezing, a chill), followed by an additional 600 mg every three hours, or 200 mg of ascorbic acid every hour. At bedtime the amount ingested is increased to 750 mg. This intake, amounting to about 4 g of ascorbic acid per day, is to be continued for three or four days, reduced to 400 mg every three hours for several days, and then to 200 mg every three hours. Dr. Régnier reported that of thirty-four colds treated with ascorbic acid plus bioflavonoids, thirty-one were averted, and of fifty colds treated with ascorbic acid alone, as described above, forty-five were averted. He had no success in treating colds with bioflavonoids alone, or with a placebo.

An important observation made by Dr. Régnier is that a cold that has been apparently aborted by the use of a large intake of ascorbic acid may return, even after a week or more, if the ingestion of ascorbic acid is suddenly discontinued.

A number of interesting comments about ascorbic acid and the common cold were made by Douglas Gildersleeve, M.D., in his article "Why Organized Medicine Sneezes at the Common Cold," published in the July—August 1967 issue of *Fact* magazine. In this article Dr. Gildersleeve* stated that "having worked as a researcher in the field, it is my contention that an effective treatment for the common cold, a cure, is available, that is being ignored because of the monetary losses that would be inflicted on pharmaceutical manufacturers, professional journals, and doctors themselves."

He wrote that he had found that he could suppress the symptoms of the common cold by making use of twenty or twenty-five times as much ascorbic acid as had been used by previous investigators, such as Tebrock, Arminio, and Johnston (Appendix III), who had used 200 mg per day. He reported that in studies carried out on more than 400 colds in twenty five individuals, mostly his own patients, he had found the treatment with ascorbic acid in large amounts to be effective in 95 percent of the patients. The most frequent cold symptom, excessive nasal discharge, disappeared entirely on use of ascorbic acid, and other symptoms, sneezing, coughing, sore throat, hoarseness, and headache, were barely noticeable, if they were present at all. He reported that not one of the subjects ever experienced any secondary bacterial complications.

Dr. Gildersleeve reported in his *Fact* article that in 1964 he wrote a paper in which he described his observations. He submitted the paper to eleven different professional journals, every one of which rejected it. Dr. Gildersleeve also reported in his *Fact* article that one editor said to him that it would be

---

*This name is probably a pseudonym, assumed by the author for professional reasons.

harmful to the journal to publish a useful treatment for the common cold. He stated that medical journals depend for their existence on the support of their advertisers, and that over twenty-five percent of the advertisements in the journals relate to patented drugs for the alleviation of cold symptoms or for the treatment of complications of colds.

Another editor said that he had rejected the paper because it was not correct. When Dr. Gildersleeve questioned him about this statement, he said, "Twenty-five years ago I was a member of a team of researchers that investigated vitamin C. We determined then that the drug was of no use in treating the common cold." He was not impressed when Dr. Gildersleeve told him that the amount of ascorbic acid that had been used in the early work was only one-twentieth of the minimum amount necessary to achieve significant results.

I think that this anecdote explains in part the slowness with which the value of ascorbic acid has been recognized by the medical profession, except as a means of preventing scurvy. Since a very small intake, about 10 mg of ascorbic acid per day, is enough to prevent scurvy from developing in most human beings, 200 mg per day seems to be a large quantity, and accordingly most of the studies that have been carried out on the possible value of ascorbic acid in controlling the common cold have been restricted to quantities of this magnitude. The possibility that the optimum rate of intake of this important food, ascorbic acid, might be much larger than 200 mg per day has been recognized only during recent years.

In April 1970 I wrote to Dr. Albert Szent-Györgyi, who is the man who had first separated ascorbic acid from the plant and animal tissues in which it occurs, and who is now in the Laboratory of the Institute for Muscle Research, Woods Hole,

Massachusetts. I asked his opinion about absorbic acid, especially with relation to the optimum rate of intake. He has given me permission to quote part of his answering letter, as follows:

> As to ascorbic acid, right from the beginning I felt that the medical profession misled the public. If you don't take ascorbic acid with your food you get scurvy, so the medical profession said that if you don't get scurvy you are all right. I think that this is a very grave error. Scurvy is not the first sign of the deficiency but a premortal syndrome, and for full health you need much more, very much more. I am taking, myself, about 1 g a day. This does not mean that this is really the optimum dose because we do not know what full health really means and how much ascorbic acid you need for it. What I can tell you is that one can take any amount of ascorbic acid without the least danger.

It may be a long time before we know what the optimum rate of intake of this important food is. There is no doubt that it varies somewhat from person to person, as discussed in Chapter 10. I am sure that an increased intake of ascorbic acid, ten to one-hundred times the daily allowance recommended by the Food and Nutrition Board, leads to improvement in general health and to increased resistance to infectious disease, including the common cold.

I am convinced by the evidence now available that ascorbic acid is to be preferred to the analgesics, antihistamines, and other dangerous drugs that are recommended for the treatment of the common cold by the purveyors of cold medicines.

Every day, even every hour, radio and television commercials extol various cold remedies. I hope that, as the results of further studies become available, extensive educational efforts about vitamin C and the common cold will be instituted on radio and television, including warnings against the use of dangerous drugs, like those about the hazards of smoking that are now sponsored by the United States Public Health Service, the American Cancer Society, the Heart Association, and other agencies.

7

Ascorbic Acid
and Influenza

The prospect of an influenza epidemic naturally leads to the question of the effectiveness of various protective measures that might be taken against influenza and related diseases. We know that the protective effect of an increased intake of ascorbic acid is not restricted to the common cold. There is, in fact, evidence that ascorbic acid significantly decreases the incidence of and mortality from so many diseases as to lead us to the conclusion that it has value in controlling essentially all diseases.

The close relation between ascorbic acid and disease is indicated by many facts. One of these facts is that epidemics of scurvy sometimes sweep through a poorly nourished populace after an epidemic of a contagious disease (Faulkner and Taylor, 1937). During the Second World War this phenomenon was observed in German prison camps (Herz, 1917). The explanation is that there is a striking decrease in the concentration of ascorbic acid in the blood plasma and cerebrospinal fluid at the onset of pneumonia, tonsillitis, rheumatic fever, acute gonorrheal arthritis, lung abscess, tuberculosis, and other diseases; the only exceptions noted in one study were uncomplicated pyelitis and cystitis (Faulkner and Taylor, 1937; Thaddea and Hoffmeister, 1937). We might accordingly conclude that patients would benefit from receiving enough ascorbic acid to make up for the decrease caused by the infection.

There is evidence that a high intake of ascorbic acid provides a considerable amount of protection against many viral diseases, probably against all. Effectiveness of ascorbic acid in inactivating the virus of poliomyelitis and protecting monkeys against paralysis after injection of the virus was reported in 1935 by Claus W. Jungeblut, who was working in the College of Physicians and Surgeons of Columbia University. He and other investigators then showed that ascorbic acid inactivates herpes virus, vaccinia virus, hepatitis virus, bacterial viruses, and other viruses (see Stone, 1972, for references). Especially thorough studies of bacterial viruses (viruses that attack bacteria) have been made by a Japanese microbiologist, Akira Murata, and his co-workers. They found that bacterial viruses of many different kinds are rendered inactive by exposure to ascorbate. Even concentrations of ascorbate in the blood as small as 3 mg per deciliter, which can be reached by a high intake of ascorbic acid by mouth or by intravenous injection of a few grams of sodium ascorbate, are effective. The rate of inactivation is greater for higher concentrations: each of the several kinds of viruses was inactivated to more than 99 percent within ten or twenty minutes by the concentration that can be reached in the blood by intravenous injection of 20 g of sodium ascorbate in an adult human being (Murata, Kitagawa, and Saruno, 1971). This direct attack on the virus by ascorbate may explain in part the effectiveness of vitamin C against viral infections, as discussed later in this chapter.

The mechanism of action has also been investigated (Murata and Kitagawa, 1973). The inactivation of the virus occurs only in the presence of free oxygen, as well as ascorbate, and it is blocked by scavengers of free radicals; that is, by molecules that destroy molecules that have an odd number of electrons. Also, the rate of inactivation is increased by even very small concentrations of copper ions (the concentrations found in blood). These facts indicate that ascorbic acid reduces the oxygen molecules to an odd-electron molecule (free radical), probably hydrogen superoxide, HO_2, which then attacks the nucleic acid of the virus.

Many reports have been published about the effectiveness of large doses of ascorbic acid in preventing and treating poliomyelitis, hepatitis, and other viral diseases. Dr. Fred R. Klenner, a physician in Reidsville, North Carolina, was the first person to report the successful treatment of polio patients by injecting large amounts of ascorbic acid (Klenner, 1949, 1951). His suggested dose for treatment of viral hepatitis is 400 to 600 mg per kilogram body weight (that is, 28 g to 42 g for a 150-pound person), repeated every eight to twelve hours, and he has administered amounts up to twice as great for various viral diseases (Klenner, 1971, 1974).

Hepatitis (called serum hepatitis) is sometimes caused in patients who receive blood transfusions by hepatitis virus in the infused blood. In some hospitals the incidence of serum hepatitis in surgical patients who are given multiple transfusions is as high as 10 percent. Dr. F. Morishige, chief surgeon in

Fukuoka General Hospital, Fukuoka, Japan, has carried out a trial that showed ascorbic acid to be thoroughly effective in protecting the patients against hepatitis. He had made an experimental study of ascorbic acid in relation to the healing of wounds while he was working for his M.D. degree, and had continued to be interested in this vitamin. He gave some of the surgical patients no vitamin C, or only a little, whereas others received large amounts. Of the 150 patients who got little or no vitamin C (less than 1.5 g per day) 11 developed serum hepatitis (incidence 7 percent), but not a single case occurred in the 1095 patients who received 2 g per day or more (Murata, 1975). Dr. Morishige now has his surgical patients and intensive-care patients take 10 g of vitamin C each day while they are in the hospital, and 6 g per day thereafter. He has also reported success with ascorbic acid in controlling other viral diseases, including measles, mumps, viral pneumonia, viral orchitis, herpes zoster (chicken pox, shingles), herpes simplex (fever blisters, cold sores), aphthous stomatitis (canker sores in the mouth), encephalomyelitis, and viral meningitis (Murata, 1975.) We may conclude from the observations reported by Klenner, Morishige, and others (twenty other references are given by Stone, 1972) that ascorbic acid has both a significant prophylactic effect and a significant therapeutic effect against all viral diseases, when it is taken in the proper amounts.

This conclusion contradicts the statements made by most medical and nutritional authorities, who continue to deny that ascorbic acid has value in protecting against viral diseases and other diseases, except scurvy. For example, in their authoritative 1,240-page treatise *Modern Nutrition in Health and Disease* (4th edition 1968) Wohl and Goodhart write that "Investigators have reported that ascorbic acid has specific therapeutic effects in a large variety of unrelated medical conditions such as rheumatic fever, rheumatoid arthritis, acute and chronic infections, allergies, intoxications, bleeding gums, peripheral vascular disease, hepatitis, and acute and chronic renal disease. These claims have not withstood the test of time." In fact, there is good evidence that ascorbic acid when taken in the proper amounts has value in controlling all of these conditions. The medical and nutritional authorities have ignored the evidence. In Chapter 12 of this book I attempt to analyze their actions and to explain their attitude.

No one has as yet carried out a thorough epidemiological study of the value of ascorbic acid in preventing influenza. There is, however, little reason to expect it to be less effective than it is with the common cold and other viral diseases. The early studies, made with a small daily intake of the vitamin, showed about the same protective effect as for the common cold. The German physician Arthur Scheunert reported in 1949 the results of a study that he had carried out with 2,600 factory workers over a period of ten months. Some of the subjects in the blind study received an inactive capsule, and others received ascorbic acid in amounts of 20, 50, 100, or 300 mg per day. The amount of protection against various illnesses, including influenza, was about the same for the groups receiving 100 mg per day and 300 mg per day, and was large, resulting in a decrease in amount of illness of 66 to 88 percent (about 20 percent for 20 mg per day and 40 percent for 50 mg per day). Scheunert concluded that the optimum intake for most of his subjects was at least 125 mg per day. His work stimulated Renker and Wegner (1954) to carry out a trial of ascorbic acid in relation to influenza. The amount of ascorbic acid used was 100 mg per day, and the study was continued for ten months. The incidence of influenza in the workers receiving ascorbic acid was only about one-quarter (28 percent) of that in the control group, and the average duration of the illness was 10 percent less. The investigators recommend that 100 mg of ascorbic acid be given to every worker each day, and point out that there would then on the average be five days less lost from work by each worker each year because of influenza, if the exposure to influenza virus were the same as during the period of their study.

Successful treatment of severe cases of influenza with large doses of ascorbic acid, as much as 24 g in twelve hours, has been reported by Klenner (1949, 1971). Albanese (1947) and Vargas Magne (1963) also obtained good results with use of a few grams per day. Use of even as small amounts as 300 mg per day has been found to reduce the length of the period of illness with influenza by 25 percent (Kimbarowski and Mokrow, 1967).

SECONDARY INFECTIONS

Influenza and pneumonia cause about sixty thousand deaths per year in the United States—many more, of course, when there is a pandemic. In some cases of death following infection with influenza, only the influenza virus is found in the lung, but often secondary bacterial infection is also present, the organisms involved being hemolytic streptococcus, staphylococcus, pneumococcus, *Hemophilus influenzae,* and *Klebsiella pneumoniae.* It is fortunate that a good intake of vitamin C provides protection not only against the viruses but also against the bacteria.

Irwin Stone (1972) has described ascorbic acid in relation to bacterial diseases in the following words:

1. It is bactericidal or bacteriostatic and will kill or prevent the growth of the pathogenic organisms.
2. It detoxicates and renders harmless the bacterial toxins and poisons.
3. It controls and maintains phagocytosis.
4. It is harmless and nontoxic and can be administered in the large doses needed to accomplish the above effects without danger to the patient.

Many investigators have reported that ascorbate inactivates bacteria. One of the earliest studies was that of Boissevin and Spillane (1937), who showed that an ascorbate concentration of 1 mg per deciliter, which is easily reached in the blood, prevents the growth of cultures of the tuberculosis bacterium. Effectiveness of ascorbate in inactivating many other bacteria and their toxins has also been reported, including the toxins of diphtheria, tetanus, staphylococcus, and dysentery, and the bacteria that cause typhoid fever, diphtheria, tetanus, and staphyloccus infections (references are given by Stone, 1972). The mechanism of the inactivation seems to be similar to that for viruses: attack by free radicals formed by ascorbate and molecular oxygen, catalyzed by copper ions (Ericsson and Lundbeck, 1955; Miller, 1969).

Klenner (1971), McCormick (1952), and others have reported a considerable degree of success in treating various bacterial infections in humans with large doses of ascorbic acid. This success may be attributed to some extent to the direct inactivation of the viruses, but I think that for the most part it results from the action of ascorbic acid in increasing the power of the natural protective mechanisms of the body (Cameron and Pauling, 1973, 1974). One of these protective mechanisms is phagocytosis, the action of white blood cells (leukocytes) in ingesting bacterial cells and destroying them. It was discovered long ago that leukocytes are not phagocytically effective if they contain only a small amount of ascorbate (Cottingham and Mills, 1943). A recent study (Hume and Weyers, 1973) has shown that persons on an ordinary Scottish diet and in good health had a little more ascorbate in their leukocytes than the amount needed for phagocytic activity, but the amount dropped to half this value on the first day after they had contracted colds, and stayed low for several days, rendering them susceptible to secondary bacterial infections. An intake of 250 mg of ascorbic acid per day was not enough to keep the amount of ascorbate in the leukocytes up to the level required for effective phagocytosis, but 1 g per day plus 6 g per day beginning at the onset of the cold was found to be enough to keep this important protective mechanism operating.

I conclude from this study that the prophylactic intake of ascorbic acid, the dose taken regularly to preserve good health and provide protection against disease, almost certainly should be more than 250 mg per day for most people. Other considerations led me to suggest the range 250 mg to 4,000 mg, or even 10,000 mg, for recommended daily intake for most people (Pauling, 1974c). Such an intake should decrease the chance of contracting the common cold or influenza and, in case that the viral infection is contracted, should prevent a secondary bacterial infection from developing. Furthermore, it is my opinion that if ascorbic acid is used in the right way in the future we shall be able to avert epidemics and pandemics of influenza.

8

Vitamin C and Evolution

A human being requires many different foods in order to be in good health. In addition to carbohydrates, proteins, essential fats, and minerals, he requires ascorbic acid and a number of other vitamins.

The protein in our diet is the principal source of the nitrogen required for the nitrogenous substances in our body, proteins and nucleic acids.

The proteins in the human body, and in other living organisms, are linear chains of residues of about twenty different amino acids—glycine, alanine, serine, lysine, phenylalanine, and fifteen others. It is not necessary that all of the amino acids be present in the diet. Some of them can be synthesized in the human body. But eight amino acids, called the essential amino acids, cannot be synthesized in the human body, and must be present in the food that is ingested. The eight essential amino acids are threonine, valine, methionine, lysine, histidine, phenylalanine, tryptophan, and leucine. The disease kwashiorkor (protein starvation) results from an inadequate intake of the essential amino acids.

We are accustomed to thinking of man as the highest of all species of living organisms. In one sense he is: he has achieved effective control over a large part of the earth, and has even begun to extend his realm as far as the moon and Mars. But in his biochemical capabilities he is inferior to many other organisms, including even unicellular organisms, such as bacteria, yeasts, and molds.

The red bread mold (*Neurospora*), for example, is able to carry out in its cells a great many chemical reactions that human beings are unable to carry out. The red bread mold can live on a very simple medium, consisting of water, inorganic salts, an inorganic source of nitrogen, such as ammonium nitrate, a suitable source of carbon, such as sucrose, and a single "vitamin," biotin. All other substances required by the red bread mold are synthesized by it, with use of its internal mechanisms. The red bread mold does not need to have any amino acids in its diet, because it is able to synthesize all of them, and also to synthesize all of the vitamins except biotin.

The red bread mold owes its survival, over hundreds of millions of years, to its great biochemical capabilities. If, like man, it were unable to synthesize the various amino acids and vitamins it would not have survived, because it could not have solved the problem of getting an adequate diet.

From time to time a gene in the red bread mold undergoes a mutation, such as to cause the cell to lose the ability to manufacture one of the amino acids or vitamin-like substances essential to its life. This mutated spore gives rise to deficient strain of red bread mold, which could stay in good health only with an addition to the diet that suffices for the original type of the mold. The scientists G. W. Beadle and E. L. Tatum carried on extensive studies of mutated strains of the red bread mold, when they were working in Stanford University, beginning about 1938. They were able to keep the mutant strains alive in the laboratory by providing each strain with the additional food that it needed for good health, as shown by a normal rate of growth.

It was mentioned in Chapter 4 that the substance thiamine (vitamin B_1) is needed by human beings to keep them from dying of the disease beriberi, and that chickens fed on a diet that contains none of this food also die of a neurological disease resembling beriberi. It has been found, in fact, that thiamine is needed as an essential food for all other animal species that have been studied, including the domestic pigeon, the laboratory rat, the guinea pig, the pig, the cow, the domestic cat, and the monkey.

We may surmise that the need of all of these animal species for thiamine as an essential food, which they must ingest in order not to develop a disease resembling beriberi in human beings, resulted from an event that took place over 500 million years ago. Let us consider the epoch, early in the history of life on earth, when the early animal species from which present-day birds and mammals have evolved populated a part of the earth. We assume that the animals of this species nourished themselves by eating plants, possibly together with other food. All plants contain thiamine. Accordingly the animals would have in their bodies the thiamine that they had ingested with the foodstuffs that they had eaten, as well as the thiamine that they themselves synthesized by use of their own synthetic mechanism. Now let us assume that a mutant animal appeared in the population, an animal that, as the result of impact of a cosmic ray on a gene or of the action of some other mutagenic agent, had lost the biochemical machinery that still permitted the other members of the species to manufacture thiamine from other substances. The amount of thiamine provided by the ingestion of food would suffice to keep the mutant well nourished, essentially as well nourished as the unmutated animals, and the mutant would have an advantage over the unmutated animals, in that it would be liberated of the burden of the machinery for manufacturing its own thiamine. As a result the mutant would be able to have more offspring than the other animals in the population. By reproduction the mutated animal would pass its advantageously mutated gene along to some of its offspring, and they too would have more than the average number of offspring. Thus in the course of time this advantage, the advantage of not having to do the work of manufacturing thiamine or to carry within itself the machinery for this manufacture, could permit the mutant type to replace the original type.

Many different kinds of molecules must be present in the body of an animal in order that the animal be in good health. Some of these molecules can be synthesized by the animal; others must be ingested as foods. If the substance is available as a food, it is advantageous to the animal species to rid itself of the burden of the machinery for synthesizing it.

It is believed that, over the millenia, the ancestors of human beings were enabled, over and over again, by the availability of certain substances as foods, including the essential amino acids and the vitamins, to simplify their own biochemical lives by shuffling off the machinery that had been needed by their ancestors for synthesizing these substances. It is evolutionary processes of this sort that gradually, over periods of millions of years, led to the appearance of new species, including man.

Some very interesting experiments have been carried out on competition between strains of organisms that require a certain substance as food and those that do not require the substance, because of the ability to synthesize it themselves. These experiments were carried out in the University of California, Los Angeles, by Zamenhof and Eichhorn, who published their findings in 1967. They studied a bacterium, *Bacillus subtilis,* by comparing a strain that had the power of manufacturing the amino acid tryptophan and a mutant strain that had lost the ability to manufacture this amino acid. If the same numbers of cells of the two strains were put in a medium that did not contain any tryptophan, the strain that could manufacture tryptophan survived, whereas the other strain died out. If, however, some cells of the two strains were put together in a medium containing a good supply of tryptophan the scales were turned: the mutant strain, which had lost the ability to manufacture the amino acid, survived, and the original strain, with the ability to manufacture the amino acid, died out. The two strains of bacteria differed only in a single mutation, the loss of the ability to manufacture the amino acid tryptophan. We are hence led to conclude that the burden of using the machinery for tryptophan synthesis was disadvantageous to the strain possessing this ability, and hampered it, in its competition with the mutant strain, to such an extent as to cause it to fail in this competition. The number of generations (cell divisions) required for take-over in this series of experiments (starting with an equal number of cells, to a million times as many cells of the victorious strain) was about fifty, which would correspond to only about fifteen hundred years for man (thirty years per generation).

We may say that Zamenhof and Eichhorn carried out a small-scale experiment about the process of the evolution of species. This experiment, and several others that they also carried out, showed that it can be advantageous to be free of the internal machinery for synthesizing a vital substance, if the vital substance can be obtained instead as a food from the immediate environment.

Most of the vitamins required by man for good health are also required by animals of other species. Vitamin A is an essential nutrient for all vertebrates for vision, maintenance of skin tissue, and normal development of bones. Riboflavin (vitamin B_2), pantothenic acid, pyridoxine (vitamin B_6), nicotinic acid (niacin), and cyanocobalamin (vitamin B_{12}) are required for good health by the cow, pig, rat, chicken, and other animals. It is likely that the loss of the ability to synthesize these essential substances, like the loss of the ability to synthesize thiamine, occurred rather early in the history of life on earth, when the primitive animals began living largely on plants, which contain a supply of these nutrients.

Irwin Stone pointed out in 1965 that, whereas most species of animals can synthesize ascorbic acid, man and other primates that have been tested, including the rhesus monkey, the Formosan long tail monkey, and the ringtail or brown capuchin monkey, are unable to synthesize the substance, and require it as a vitamin. He concluded that the loss of the ability to synthesize ascorbic acid probably occurred in the common ancestor of the primates. A rough estimate of the time at which this mutational change occurred is 25 million years ago (Zuckerkandl and Pauling, 1962).

The guinea pig and an Indian fruit-eating bat are the only other mammals known to require ascorbic acid as a vitamin. The red-vented bulbul and some other Indian birds (of the order Passeriformes) also require ascorbic acid. The overwhelming majority of mammals, birds, amphibians, and reptiles have the ability to synthesize the substance in their tissues, usually in the liver or the kidney. The loss of the ability by the guinea pig, the fruit-eating bat, and the red-vented bulbul and some other species of passeriform birds probably resulted from independent mutations in populations of these species of animals living in an environment that provided an ample supply of ascorbic acid in the available foodstuffs.

We may ask why ascorbic acid is not required as a vitamin in the food of the cow, pig, horse, rat, chicken, and many other species of animals that do require the other vitamins required by man. Ascorbic acid is present in green plants, along with these other vitamins. When green plants became the steady diet of the common ancestor of man and other mammals, hundreds of millions of years ago, why did not this ancestor undergo the mutation of eliminating the mechanism for synthesizing ascorbic acid, as well as the mechanisms for synthesizing thiamine, pantothenic acid, pyridoxine, and other vitamins?

I think that the answer to this question is that for optimum health more ascorbic acid was needed than could be provided under ordinary conditions by the usually available green plants.

Let us consider the common precursor of the primates, at a time about 25 million years ago. This animal and his ancestors had for hundreds of millions of years continued to synthesize ascorbic acid from other substances that they had ingested. Let us assume that a population of this species of animals was living, at that time, in an area that provided an ample supply of food with an unusually large content of ascorbic acid, permitting the animals to obtain from their diet approximately the amount of ascorbic acid needed for optimum health. A cosmic ray or some other mutagenic agent then caused a mutation to occur, such that the enzyme in the liver that catalyzes the conversion of L-gulonolactone to ascorbic acid was no longer present in the liver. Some of the progeny of this mutant animal would have inherited the loss of the ability to synthesize ascorbic acid. These mutant animals would, in the environment that provided an ample supply of ascorbic acid, have an advantage over the ascorbic-acid-producing animals, in that they had been relieved of the burden of constructing and operating the machinery for producing ascorbic acid. Under these conditions the mutant would gradually replace the earlier strain.

A mutation that involves the loss of the ability to synthesize an enzyme occurs often. Such a mutation requires only that the gene be damaged in some way or be deleted. (The reverse mutation, leading to the ability to produce the enzyme, is difficult, and would occur only extremely rarely). Once the ability to synthesize ascorbic acid has been lost by a species of animals, that species depends for its existence on the availability of ascorbic acid as a food.

The fact that most species of animals have not lost the ability to manufacture their own ascorbic acid shows that the supply

of ascorbic acid available generally in foodstuffs is not sufficient to provide the optimum amount of this substance. Only
in an unusual environment, in which the available food
provided unusually large amounts of ascorbic acid, have
circumstances permitted a species of animal to abandon its
own powers of synthesis of this important substance. These
unusual circumstances occurred for the precursor of man and
other primates, for the guinea pig, for the Indian fruit-eating
bat, and for the precursor of the red-vented bulbul and some
other species of passeriform birds, but have not occurred,
through the hundreds of millions of years of evolution, for the
precursors of the cow, the horse, the pig, the rat, and hundreds
of other animals. Thus the consideration of evolutionary
processes, as presented in the foregoing analysis, indicates that
the ordinarily available foodstuffs might well provide essentially the optimum amounts of thiamine, riboflavin, niacin,
vitamin A, and other vitamins that are required as essential
nutrients by all mammalian species, but be deficient in
ascorbic acid. For this food, essential for man but synthesized
by many other species of animals, the optimum rate of intake is
indicated to be larger than the rate associated with the
ingestion of the ordinarily available diet.

I have checked the amounts of various vitamins present in
110 raw, natural plant foods, as given in the tables in the
metabolism handbook published by the Federation of American Societies for Experimental Biology (Altman and Dittmer,
1968). When the amounts of vitamins corresponding to one
day's food for an adult (the amount that provides 2,500
kilocalories of energy) are calculated, it is found that for most
vitamins this amount is about three times the daily allowance
recommended by the Food and Nutrition Board. For ascorbic

acid, however, the average amount in the daily ration of the 110 plant foodstuffs is 2.3 g, about fifty-one times the amount recommended as the daily allowance for a person with a caloric requirement of 2,500 kilocalories per day (see Table 3.)

If the need for ascorbic acid were really as small as the daily allowance recommended by the Food and Nutrition Board the mutation would surely have occurred 500 million years ago, and dogs, cows, pigs, horses, and other animals would be obtaining ascorbic acid from their food, instead of manufacturing it in their own liver cells.

Therefore, I conclude that 2.3 g per day is less than the optimum rate of intake of ascorbic acid for an adult human being.

The average ascorbic-acid content of the fourteen plant food-stuffs richest in this vitamin is 9.4 g per 2,500 kilocalories. Peppers (hot or sweet, green or red) and black currants are riches of all, with 15 g per 2,500 kilocalories. These amounts indicate an upper limit for the optimum daily intake for man.

I conclude that the optimum daily intake of ascorbic acid for most adult human beings lies in the range 2.3 g to 9 g. The amount of individual biochemical variability (Chapter 10) is such that for a large population the range may be as great as from 250 mg to 10 g or more per day.

The foregoing argument represents an extension and refinement of arguments advanced by the biochemists G. H. Bourne and Irwin Stone. In 1949 Bourne pointed out that the food ingested by the gorilla consists largely of fresh vegetation, in quantity such as to give the gorilla about 4.5 of ascorbic acid per day, and that before the development of agriculture man existed largely on green plants, supplemented with some meat. He concluded that "it may be possible, therefore, that when we

TABLE 3
Vitamin content of 110 raw natural plant foods referred to the amount giving 2,500 kilocalories of food energy

Foods	Thiamine	Riboflavin	Niacin	Ascorbic acid
Nuts and grains (11)	3.2 mg	1.5 mg	27 mg	0 mg
Fruit, low C (21)	1.9	2.0	19	600
Beans and peas (15)	7.5	4.7	34	1,000
Berries, low C (8)	1.7	2.0	15	1,200
Vegetables, low C (25)	5.0	5.9	39	1,200
Intermediate-C foods (16)	7.8	9.8	77	3,400
High-C foods (6)	8.1	19.6	58	6,000
Very high-C foods (8)	6.1	9.0	68	12,000
Averages for 110 foods	5.0	5.4	41	2,300
Recommended daily allowance for male adult	1.5 mg	1.6 mg	18 mg	45 mg
Ratio of plant food average to average recommended allowance	3.3	3.4	2.3	51

Nuts and grains: almonds, filberts, macadamia nuts, peanuts, barley, brown rice, whole grain rice, sesame seeds, sunflower seeds, wheat, wild rice.

Fruit (low in vitamin C, less than 2,500 mg): apples, apricots, avocadoes, bananas, cherries (sour red, sweet), coconut, dates, figs, grapefruit, grapes, kumquats, mangoes, nectarines, peaches, pears, pineapple, plums, crabapples, honeydew melon, watermelon.

Beans and peas: broad beans (immature seeds, mature seeds), cowpeas (immature seeds, mature seeds), lima beans (immature seeds, mature seeds), mung beans (seeds, sprouts), peas (edible pod, green mature seeds), snapbeans (green, yellow), soybeans (immature seeds, mature seeds, sprouts).

Berries (low C, less than 2,500 mg): blackberries, blueberries, cranberries, loganberries, raspberries, currants (red), gooseberries, tangerines.

Vegetables (low C, less than 2,500 mg): bamboo shoots, beets, carrots, celeriac root, celery, corn, cucumber, dandelion greens, egg-plant, garlic cloves, horseradish, lettuce, okra, onions (young, mature), parsnips, potatoes, pumpkins, rhubarb, rutabagas, squash (summer, winter), sweet potatoes, green tomatoes, yams.

Intermediate-C foods (2,500 to 4,900 mg): artichokes, asparagus, beet greens, cantaloupe, chicory greens, chinese cabbage, fennel, lemons, limes, oranges, radishes, spinach, zucchini, strawberries, swiss chard, ripe tomatoes.

High-C foods (5,000 to 7,900 mg): brussels sprouts, cabbage, cauliflower, chives, collards, mustard greens.

Very high-C foods (8,000 to 16,500 mg): broccoli spears, black currants, kale, parsley, hot chili peppers (green, red), sweet peppers (green, red).

are arguing whether 7 or 30 mg of vitamin C a day is an adequate intake we may be very wide of the mark. Perhaps we should be arguing whether 1 g or 2 g a day is the correct amount." Stone (1966a) quoted this argument, and supplemented it by consideration of the rate of manufacture of ascorbic acid by the rat. The rat under normal conditions is reported to synthesize ascorbic acid at a rate between 26 mg per day per kilogram of body weight (Burns, Mosbach, and Schulenberg, 1954) and 58 mg per day kilogram of body weight (Salomon and Stubbs, 1961). If the assumption is made that the same rate of production would be proper for a human being, a person weighing 70 kg (154 pounds) should ingest between 1.8 g and 4.1 g per day under ordinary circumstances. Other animals, including the goat, cow, sheep, mouse, squirrel, gerbil, rabbit, cat, and dog, also manufacture ascorbic acid at a high rate, averaging about 10 g per day for 70 kg (154 pounds) body weight (Chatterjee and others, 1975). It is hard to believe that these animals would make this large amount of ascorbic acid if it were not beneficial to them, and also hard to believe that man is so much different from other animals that he can keep in the best of health with only one two-hundredth of the amounts that they use.

In general, the dietary requirements of man have been found to be closely similar to those of other primates, and studies of vitamin C in these primates should yield valuable information about the optimum intake of this vitamin. Monkeys are used in large numbers in medical research, and much effort has been devoted to finding the intakes of various nutrients that puts them in the best of health (Subcommittee on Laboratory Animal Nutrition, 1972). These careful studies have led to the formulation of several rather similar recommended diets for laboratory monkeys. The amount of ascorbic acid in these diets lies in the range of 1.75 g per day to 3.50 g per day, calculated to 70 kg body weight; for example, 1.75 g per day for rhesus monkeys (Rinehart and Greenberg, 1956) and 3.50 g per day for squirrel monkeys (Portman et al., 1967). (These monkeys weigh only a few kilograms, but there is little doubt that the need for ascorbic acid is proportional to body weight, because the amounts manufactured by different animals that have the ability to make this substance are found to be rather closely proportional to body weight over a tremendous range, from a 20-g mouse to a 70-kg goat.) From these studies with monkeys we may conclude that the optimum intake of vitamin C by man probably also lies in the range of 1.75 g to 3.50 g per day, in agreement with the conclusion reached from other arguments.

Additional evidence has been provided by a study of the optimum intake of ascorbic acid by guinea pigs. Yew (1973) found that observations of growth rates both before and after surgical stress, recovery times after anesthesia, scab formation, wound healing, and the production of hydroxyproline and hydroxylysine during wound healing all support the conclusion that young guinea pigs ordinarily need about 5.0 mg per 100 g of body weight per day, and that under stress the needs are even higher. For man the corresponding intake is 3.5 g per day under ordinary conditions, a larger amount under stress.

Why have not similar studies been carried out with human beings? Part of the answer is that it is much harder to carry out studies with human beings than with animals. Another part is that many physicians and nutritionists seem to have accepted the idea that vitamin C has no value for human beings except to prevent scurvy, and that it would be a waste of effort to attempt to determine the optimum intake. Still another aspect of this matter is that in fact many studies have been carried out that indicate that an intake of several grams per day leads to improved health; these studies are described in this book.

It is almost certain that some evolutionarily effective mutations have occurred in man and his immediate predecessors rather recently (within the last few million years) such as to permit life to continue on an intake of ascorbic acid less than that provided by high-ascorbic-acid raw plant foods. These mutations might involve an increased ability of the kidney tubules to pump ascorbic acid back into the blood from the glomerular filtrate (dilute urine, being concentrated on passage along the tubules) and an increased ability of certain cells to extract ascorbic acid from the blood plasma. It is likely that the adrenal glands act as a storehouse of ascorbic acid, extracting it from the blood when green plant foods are available, in the summer, and releasing it slowly when the supply is depleted. On general principles we can conclude, however, that these mechanisms require energy and are a burden to the organism. The optimum rate of intake of ascorbic acid might still be within the range given above, 2.3 g per day or more, or might be somewhat less; and, of course, there is always the factor of biochemical individuality, discussed in Chapter 10.

9

Orthomolecular Medicine

Orthomolecular medicine is the preservation of good health and the treatment of disease by varying the concentrations in the human body of substances that are normally present in the body and are required for health (Pauling, 1968b).

Death by starvation, kwashiorkor, beriberi, scurvy, or any other deficiency disease can be averted by the provision of an adequate daily intake of carbohydrates, essential fats, proteins (including the essential amino acids), essential minerals, thiamine, ascorbic acid, and other vitamins. To achieve the best of health, the rate of intake of essential foods should be such as to establish and maintain the optimum concentrations of essential molecules, such as those of ascorbic acid. There is no doubt that a high concentration of ascorbic acid is needed to provide the maximum protection against infection, and to permit the rapid healing of wounds. I believe that in general the treatment of disease by the use of substances, such as ascorbic acid, that are normally present in the human body and are required for life is to be preferred to the treatment by the use of powerful synthetic substances or plant products, which may, and usually do, have undesirable side effects.

An example of orthomolecular medicine is the treatment of diabetes mellitus by the injection of insulin. Diabetes mellitus is a hereditary disease, usually caused by a recessive gene. The hereditary defect results in a deficient production by the pancreas of the hormone insulin. The primary effect of insulin is to cause an increase in the rate of extraction of glucose from the blood. In the absence of insulin the concentration of glucose in the blood of the patient becomes much greater than normal, resulting in the manifestations of the disease.

Insulin extracted from cattle pancreas or pig pancreas differs only slightly in its molecular structure from human insulin, and it has essentially the same physiological activity. The injection of cattle insulin or pig insulin is essentially the provision of the normal concentration of insulin in the body of the patient; it permits the metabolism of glucose to take place at the normal rate, and thus serves to counteract the abnormality resulting from the genetic defect. Insulin therapy is accordingly an example of orthomolecular therapy. Its major disadvantage is that the insulin cannot be introduced into the blood stream except by injection.

Another way in which the disease can be kept under control, if it is not serious, is by adjusting the diet, regulating the intake of sugar, in such a way as to keep the glucose concentration in the blood within the normal limits. This procedure also represents an example of orthomolecular medicine. Another example is the use of an increased intake of vitamin C to decrease the need for insulin. Dice and Daniel (1973) reported from the study of one diabetic subject that for each gram of L-ascorbic acid taken by mouth the amount of insulin required could be reduced by two units.

A fourth procedure, the use of so-called oral insulin, a drug taken by mouth, does not constitute an example of orthomolecular medicine, because oral insulin is a synthetic drug, foreign to the human body, that may have undesirable side effects.

Another disease that is treated by orthomolecular methods is phenylketonuria. Phenylketonuria results from a genetic defect that leads to a decreased amount of effectiveness of an enzyme in the liver which in normal persons catalyzes the oxidation of one amino acid, phenylalanine, to another, tyrosine. Ordinary proteins contain several percent of phenylalanine, providing a much larger amount of this amino acid than a person needs. The concentration of phenylalanine in the blood and other body fluids of the patient becomes abnormally high, if he is on a normal diet, causing the manifestations of the disease: mental deficiency, severe eczema, and others. The disease can be controlled by use, beginning in infancy, of a diet that contains a smaller amount of phenylalanine than is present in ordinary foods. In this way the concentration of phenylalanine in the blood and other body fluids is kept to approximately the normal level, and the manifestations of the disease do not appear.

A somewhat similar disease, which can also be controlled by orthomolecular methods, is galactosemia. Galactosemia involves the failure to manufacture an enzyme that carries out the metabolism of galactose, which is a part of milk sugar (lactose). The disease manifests itself in mental retardation, cataracts, cirrhosis of the liver and spleen, and nutritional failure. These manifestations are averted by placing the infant on a diet free of milk sugar, with the result that the concentration of galactose in the blood does not exceed the normal limit.

A conceivable sort of orthomolecular therapy for a hereditary disease involving a defective gene would be to introduce the gene (molecules of DNA, deoxyribonucleic acid), separated from the tissues of another person, into the cells of the person suffering from the disease. For example, some molecules of the gene that directs the synthesis of the enzyme that catalyzes the oxidation of phenylalanine to tyrosine could be separated from liver cells of a normal human being and introduced into the liver cells of a person with phenylketonuria. This sort of change in genetic character of an organism has been carried out for microorganisms, but not yet for human beings, and it is not likely that it will become an important way of controlling genetic defects until many decades have passed.

Another possible method of orthomolecular therapy for phenylketonuria, resembling the use of insulin in controlling diabetes, would be the injection of the active enzyme. There are two reasons why this treatment has not been developed. First, although it is known that the enzyme is present in the liver of animals, including man, it has not yet been isolated in purified form. Second, the natural mechanism of immunity, which involves the action of antibodies against proteins foreign to the species, would operate to destroy the enzyme prepared from the liver of animals of another species. This mechanism in general prevents the use of enzymes or other proteins from animals other than man in the treatment of diseases of human beings. Insulin is an exceptional protein, in that the molecules are unusually small. The insulin molecule contains polypeptide chains of two kinds, one containing 21 amino-acid residues and the other containing 30, whereas the polypeptide chains of most proteins contain between 100 and 200 residues. The structural difference between human insulin and animal insulin is very small; for example, pig insulin differs from human insulin in only one residue of the total of 51. This difference is so small as not to invoke the production of antibodies.

There is still another possible type of orthomolecular therapy. The molecules of many enzymes consist of two parts: the pure protein part, called the apoenzyme, and a non-protein part, called the coenzyme. The active enzyme, called the holo-enzyme, is the apoenzyme with the coenzyme attached to it. Often the coenzyme is a vitamin molecule or a closely related molecule. It is known, for example, that a number of different enzymes in the human body, catalyzing different chemical reactions, have thiamine diphosphate, a derivative of thiamine (vitamin B_1), as coenzyme.

In some cases of genetic disease the enzyme is not absent, but is present with diminished activity. One way in which the defective gene can operate is to produce an apoenzyme with abnormal structure, such that it does not combine readily with the coenzyme to form the active enzyme. Under ordinary physiological conditions, with the normal concentration of coenzyme, perhaps only one percent of the abnormal apoenzyme has combined with the coenzyme. According to the principles of chemical equilibrium, a larger fraction of the abnormal apoenzyme could be made to combine with the coenzyme by increasing the concentration of the coenzyme in the body fluids. If the concentration were to be increased one hundred times, most of the apoenzyme molecules might combine with the coenzyme, to give essentially the normal amount of active enzyme.

There is accordingly the possibility that the disease could be kept under control by the ingestion by the patient of a very large amount of the vitamin that serves as a coenzyme. This sort of orthomolecular therapy, involving only a substance normally present in the human body (the vitamin), is, in my opinion, the preferable therapy.

An example of a disease that might be controlled in this way is the disease methylmalonicaciduria. The patients with this disease are deficient in the active enzyme that catalyzes the conversion of a simple substance, methylmalonic acid, to succinic acid. It is known that cyanocobalamin (vitamin B_{12}) serves as the coenzyme for this reaction. It is found that the provision of very large amounts of vitamin B_{12}, giving concentrations about a thousand times the normal concentration, causes the reaction to proceed at the normal rate for many patients.

The use of very large amounts of vitamins in the control of disease has been called megavitamin therapy. Megavitamin therapy is one aspect of orthomolecular medicine. It is my opinion that in the course of time it will be found possible to control hundreds of diseases by megavitamin therapy. For example, Dr. A. Hoffer and Dr. H. Osmond have reported that many patients with schizophrenia are benefited by megavitamin therapy (Hoffer, 1962; Hoffer and Osmond, 1966). Their treatment, as was mentioned in the Introduction, includes the administration of nicotinic acid (niacin) or nicotinamide (niacinamide) in amounts of 3 g to 18 g per day, together with 3 g to 18 g per day of ascorbic acid, and good amounts of other vitamins (Hawkins and Pauling, 1973; Pauling, 1974b).

It is usually thought that a drug that is claimed to be a cure for many different diseases cannot have any value against any one of them. Yet there is evidence, summarized in this book, that a large intake of vitamin C helps to control a great many diseases: not only the common cold and the flu, but also other viral and bacterial diseases, such as hepatitis, and also quite unrelated diseases, including schizophrenia, cardiovascular disease, and cancer. There is a reason for this difference between vitamin C and ordinary drugs. Most drugs are powerful substances that interact in a specific way with one kind of molecule or tissue or agent of disease in the body so as to help to control a particular disease. The substance may, however, interact in a harmful way with other parts of the body, thus producing the side effects that make drugs dangerous. Vitamin C, on the other hand, is a normal constituent of the body, required for life. It is involved in essentially all of the biochemical reactions that take place in the body and in all of the body's protective mechanisms. With the ordinary intake of vitamin C these reactions and mechanisms do not operate efficiently; the person ingesting only the recommended daily amount of 45 mg is in what might be called ordinary poor health—what the physicians and nutritionists call "ordinary good health." The optimum intake of vitamin C, together with other health measures, can provide *really* good health, with increased protection against all diseases.

We have been slow to recognize the value of vitamin C and other vitamins. In 1937 Szent-Györgyi wrote that "Vitamins, if properly understood and applied, will help us to reduce human suffering to an extent which the most fantastic mind would fail to imagine." Only now, forty years later, are we beginning to accept this idea.

A large rate of intake of ascorbic acid is required for optimal protection against infectious disease. The use of ascorbic acid to provide protection against the common cold, influenza, rheumatic fever, pneumonia, and other infectious diseases may well be the most important of all methods of orthomolec ular medicine.

10

Human Biochemical Individuality

In considering the problem of protection against the common cold and other diseases we must recognize that human beings differ from one another. Professor Roger J. Williams, who for many years has been interested in the question of these differences (see his books *You Are Extraordinary*, 1967; *Biochemical Individuality*, 1973; and *Physicians' Handbook of Nutritional Science*, 1975) has pointed out that it is unlikely that any human being is exactly the "average" man.

Let us consider some character, such as the weight of the liver relative to the total weight of the human being, or the concentration of a certain enzyme in the red cells of the blood. It is found that, when a sample of 100 human beings is studied, this character varies over a several-fold range. The variation often is approximately that given by the standard bell-shaped probability function. It is customary to say that the "normal" range of values of the character is that range within which 95 percent of the values lie, and that the remaining 5 percent of the values, representing the extremes, are abnormal. If we assume that 500 characters are independently inherited, then we can calculate that there is only a small chance, 10 percent, that one person in the whole population of the world would be normal with respect to each of these 500 characters. But it is estimated that a human being has a complement of 100,000 genes, each of which serves some function, such as controlling the synthesis of an enzyme. The number of characters that can be variable, because of a difference in the nature of a particular gene, is presumably somewhere near 100,000, rather than only 500; and accordingly we reach the conclusion that no single human being on earth is normal (within the range that includes 95 percent of human beings) with respect to all characters. This calculation is, of course, oversimplified; but, as mentioned by Williams, it helps emphasize the point that human beings differ from one another, and that each human being must be treated as an individual.

The species Man is more heterogeneous, with respect to genetic character, than most other animal species. Nevertheless, heterogeneity has been found also for laboratory animals such as guinea pigs. It was recognized long ago that guinea pigs fed the same scurvy-producing diet, containing less than 5 mg of ascorbic acid per day kilogram of body weight, differed in the severity of the scurvy that they developed and in the rapidity with which they developed it. A striking experiment was carried out in 1967 by Williams and Deason. These investigators obtained some male weanling guinea pigs from an animal dealer and, after a week of observation during which the guinea pigs were on a good diet, including fresh vegetables, they were placed on a diet free of ascorbic acid or with known amounts added. They were divided into eight groups, each of ten to fifteen guinea pigs, with one of the groups receiving no ascorbic acid and the other groups receiving varying amounts of ascorbic acid by mouth, given by pipet. About 80 percent of the animals receiving no ascorbic acid or only 0.5 mg per kilogram per day developed signs of scurvy, whereas only about 25 percent of those receiving between 1 mg and 4 mg per kilogram per day, and none of those receiving 8 mg per day or more, developed these signs. These results agree with the customary statement that about 5 mg per kilogram per day of ascorbic acid is required to prevent scurvy in guinea pigs.

It was observed, however, that two animals receiving only 1 mg per kilogram per day remained healthy and gained weight over the entire period of the experiment (eight weeks). One of them showed a total gain in weight larger than that for any animal receiving two, four, eight, or sixteen times as much ascorbic acid.

On the other hand, seven of the guinea pigs receiving 8, 16, or 32 mg per kilogram per day were unhealthy, and showed very small growth during the first ten days on the diet. They were then provided with a larger amount of the vitamin, five of them with 64 mg per kilogram per day and two of them with 128 mg per kilogram per day. These animals showed a remarkable response: whereas they had grown only 12 grams, on the average, in a period of ten days on the smaller amounts of ascorbic acid, their growth during the ten-day period after beginning to receive the larger amounts was, on the average, 72 grams. The indicated conclusion is that these animals, seven of the thirty that were placed on between 8 mg and 32 mg per kilogram per day, had a larger requirement of vitamin C for good health than the others. Williams and Deason reached the conclusion that there is at least a twenty-fold range in the vitamin-C needs of individual guinea pigs in a population of 100. They pointed out that the population of human beings is presumably not more uniform than that of the guinea pigs used in their experiments, and that accordingly the individual variation in human vitamin C needs is probably just as great.

I have accepted their conclusion, and similar conclusions reached by other investigators, in suggesting that the optimum rate of intake of ascorbic acid by human beings may extend over a wide range, perhaps the forty-fold range from 250 mg per day to 10 g per day or an even wider range.

Vitamin C was first isolated nearly fifty years ago, and many thousands of scientific papers have been published in which the results of studies of it are reported. The reader of this book might well be justified in asking why the range of values of the optimum intake of this important substance was not reliably determined long ago, and also how he can find out what amount he himself should take to be in the best of health. Part of the answer to the first question is that only a very small amount of the vitamin, perhaps 10 mg per day, is enough to keep most people from developing scurvy, and physicians and nutritionists accepted the idea that no larger amount is needed. Even though some physicians had observed thirty or forty years ago that amounts a hundred or a thousand times larger have value in controlling various diseases, as described earlier in this book, the medical profession and most scientists ignored the evidence. Another part of the answer to this question is that studies that would yield the answer can be carried out only with great effort and at great expense. It is much easier to investigate some powerful drug that has an immediate beneficial effect on the patient (although it is harder to check the possible long-term damage that the powerful drug may do to some fraction of the people for whom it is prescribed). Several excellently planned and executed epidemiological studies involving nutritional factors and other factors in relation to the incidence of disease and the chance of death at various ages have been carried out. In some of these studies the nature of the ingested food has been tabulated, and the amounts of vitamin C and other vitamins in the diet have been calculated with use of tables giving the vitamin contents of various foods. Some of these studies show that the incidence of disease and the chance of death at each age are less for people with a larger intake of vitamin C (and also for some other vitamins) than for those with a smaller intake. In these studies, however, the intakes of vitamin C are small; for example, 0 mg to 50 mg per day for the low-intake group and more than 50 mg (an average of about 100 mg) for the high-intake group.

The results of one of these epidemiological studies, carried out in San Mateo County, California, were reported by Chope and Breslow (1956), and Drake et al., (1957). In 1948 they and their collaborators interviewed 577 randomly selected residents of the county who were fifty years old or older. They obtained much information about their state of health and about environmental, behavioral, and nutritional factors that might affect it. After seven years they examined the death records and compared the age-corrected death rates for the subpopulations related to the different factors. Of all of these factors, the intake of vitamin C was found to have the greatest correlation with the age-corrected death rate, even greater than that for cigarette smoking. Whereas cigarette smokers have at each age twice the chance of dying that a nonsmoker has, the persons with a lower intake of vitamin C (calculated from the content of vitamin C in the food that they ate) had a chance of dying 2.5 times greater than the persons with a higher intake of the vitamin. The amount of illness was also correspondingly greater. This difference means that the length of the period of good health and of life was ten years greater for the persons with the higher intake than for those with the lower intake of vitamin C. The dividing line was 50 mg per day, approximately equal to the recommended dietary allowance (45 mg per day). The average intake of the low-C group was 24 mg per day and that of the high-C group was 127 mg per day.* It is interesting that drinking a large glass of orange juice each day (about 90 mg of ascorbic acid in 6 ounces of juice) or taking a 100-mg tablet each day would put a person in the high-C group.

Part of the improvement in health of the high-C group may be attributed to other substances in the foods that provided the extra vitamin C. There is no doubt that orange juice, lettuce and other vegetables, and fruits contain important nutrients in addition to vitamin C. But the effect of a higher intake of vitamin A in improving the health was found in the San Mateo study to be only half as great as that of vitamin C, and that of niacin, one of the B vitamins, was only one-quarter as great. The foods with a high content of vitamin A and niacin, although they have value in improving the health, are not so valuable as those with a high content of vitamin C.

---

*These averages are calculated on the assumption that the distribution of intakes for each of the two groups is the same as for the corresponding groups (age over sixty) in the First Health and Nutrition Examination Survey, 1971–1972 (Abraham, Lowenstein, and Johnson, 1976).

WHAT HAPPENS TO VITAMIN C IN THE BODY?

When vitamin C is taken by mouth most of it is absorbed into the blood through the mucous membranes of the mouth, the stomach, and the upper part of the small intestine. If the amount taken is rather small, up to 250 mg, about 80 percent is absorbed into the blood. With larger doses the fraction absorbed is less, about 50 percent for a dose of 2 g and still smaller for larger doses (Kubler and Gehler, 1970). Accordingly it is more economical to ingest ascorbic acid in smaller doses, such as 1 g every three hours, than to take a single much larger dose once a day. Also, a few grams of sodium ascorbate injected into the blood stream is more effective in the treatment of disease than the same amount taken by mouth.

For a small daily intake of ascorbic acid, up to about 150 mg, the concentration in the blood plasma is nearly proportional to the intake: this concentration is about 5 mg per liter for a daily intake of 50 mg, 10 mg per liter for 100 mg, and 15 mg per liter for 150 mg. Above an intake of 150 mg per day the concentration in the blood increases much less with increasing intake, reaching about 30 mg per liter for an intake of 10 g per day (ascorbic acid plus dehydroascorbic acid; Harris, Robinson, and Pauling, 1973).

The reason for this change when the intake exceeds about 150 mg per day is that a larger amount of the vitamin then begins to be excreted in the urine. One of the functions of the kidney is to clear the blood of unwanted and harmful molecules, the molecules of toxic substances that have got into the blood through the food or impure air or of waste products such as urea, the compound of nitrogen that is formed when old protein molecules in the body are degraded. Every twenty minutes the entire volume of the blood passes by a set of molecular filters in the two million glomeruli of the kidney. In the glomeruli the capillaries through which the blood is flowing have small holes in them. These holes, the pores of the glomerular filter, are small enough that the protein molecules in the blood, such as the antibodies (globulins) that protect us against disease, cannot pass through them, but water molecules and other small molecules, such as those of blood sugar (glucose) and ascorbic acid, can pass through. The blood pressure operates to push part of the water of the blood, together with its burden of small molecules, through these pores into a surrounding capsule.* The glomerular filtrate, which is dilute urine, is produced in amounts of about 180 liters per day, thirty-six times the volume of the blood itself. We cannot stand to lose so much water, and fortunately there is a mechanism to concentrate the urine to the usual volume of one or two liters a day. As the glomerular filtrate moves along through tubules toward the vessels that carry the urine to the bladder, molecular pumps in the walls of the tubules transfer most of the water back into the blood stream.** The blood sugar is valuable as a fuel for the body, and it would not be good to lose it. Accordingly, there are special tubular pumps to pump the glucose molecules back into the blood. There are also

---

*A seriously ill person or a person in shock may have such low blood pressure that he cannot produce any urine.

**The process of concentrating the urine is regulated by the antidiuretic hormone, which is secreted by the pituitary gland. Some people develop a rather rare illness, diabetes insipidus, involving an insufficient output of this hormone; their urine volume may reach 40 liters per day, requiring them to drink an equal amount of water.

special pumps for other important molecules, including those of vitamin C. This is fortunate, because if the process of tubular reabsorption of vitamin C did not operate even a big dose of the vitamin would be nearly completely excreted in an hour or two. In fact, a person who ingests 100 mg per day excretes only about 10 mg in his urine.

The necessity of conserving our supply of ascorbic acid arose when our ancestors lost the ability to synthesize it and we were required to depend on what we could get in our food. We have developed the mechanism of tubular reabsorption to such an extent that it works nearly perfectly (pumping 99.5 percent of the ascorbate in the glomerular filtrate back into the blood stream) until it reaches the limit of its pumping capacity. This limit is reached when the concentration in the blood plasma equals about 14 mg per liter, corresponding to a daily intake of about 140 mg.

When the discovery was made that at higher intakes than 140 mg per day a greatly increased amount of vitamin C is excreted in the urine the idea was developed that at 140 mg per day the tissues of the body are saturated with the vitamin and are beginning to reject any additional amount. Although this idea is false, it continues to be advanced in the medical and nutritional literature, and the intake of 140 mg per day, corresponding to the so-called "tissue saturation," is considered to be an upper limit to the amount of vitamin C required for "ordinary good health."

An argument similar to those developed in Chapter 8, on the other hand, leads us to the conclusion that this intake, at which the tubular pumps reach their capacity, is a *lower* limit to the optimum intake (Pauling, 1974). Let us compare a tubular pump for ascorbic acid that operates up to 14 mg per liter with one that operates only to 13 mg per liter. The smaller pump is 7 percent smaller than the other and requires 7 percent less energy, which is provided by the food that we burn as fuel, for its operation. The smaller pump would accordingly be less of a burden to us than the larger one. Then why should we have developed the larger pump? The answer surely is that we need the larger pump to conserve the extra 7 percent of vitamin C. Hence the limit to which tubular reabsorption has been developed represents a lower limit to the optimum intake of vitamin C.

This lower limit is three times the recommended daily allowance set by the U.S. Food and Nutrition Board.

If a large amount of vitamin C is taken, 62 percent of the amount that gets into the blood stream is excreted in the urine, so that only about 38 percent remains in the body to carry on its valuable functions. It is, in fact, good to have vitamin C in the urine. It protects against urinary infections, and also against cancer of the bladder, as was mentioned in Chapter 5.

Moreover, that fraction of a large dose of vitamin C taken by mouth that remains in the intestines has value. DeCosse and his co-workers studied the effect of 3 g per day of ascorbic acid in controlling the growth of adenomatous polyps of the rectum in people who have inherited the tendency to develop them (1975). This polyposis is serious because the polyps usually develop into a malignant cancer. In the group of eight patients, the polyps regressed completely in two and partially in three.

The appearance of vitamin C in the urine has been used by nutritional authorities as an argument against a high intake. Dr. Fredrick J. Stare in his book *Eating for Good Health* (1969) states that 60 mg or 70 mg per day is enough: "an extra amount of the vitamin cannot be stored in the body and is simply excreted. You don't need vitamin-C pills under normal circumstances." These statements are repeated by him in his latest book, *Panic in the Pantry* (Whelan and Stare, 1975). He does not mention that much of a large dose is retained in the body.

The observations that have been made on the concentration of ascorbate in the blood plasma corresponding to the capacity of the mechanism of tubular reabsorption in different people give some information about biochemical individuality with respect to vitamin C. In one study, with nineteen subjects, the capacity varied between 10 mg and 20 mg per liter (Friedman, Sherry, and Ralli, 1940). Similar variation has been found by other investigators.

Ascorbic acid is present in the various body fluids and organs, especially the leukocytes and the blood. Its concentration in the brain is also high. When a person with an insufficient supply of ascorbic acid ingests a quantity of it, it moves very rapidly from the blood serum into the leukocytes, other cells, and organs such as the spleen. The amount remaining in the blood serum may be so small, less than the capacity of the mechanism of tubular reabsorption, that very little is eliminated in the urine. A test was developed long ago (Harris and Ray, 1935) to show the avidity with which the tissues remove ascorbate from the blood serum. This test, called a loading test, involves giving the subject a certain amount of the vitamin by mouth or by injection, collecting the urine for the following six hours, and analyzing it for ascorbic acid. If an oral dose of about 1 g is given, most people whose blood serum is not depleted of the vitamin eliminate about 20 or 25 percent of it in the urine in six hours.

A person who eliminates a smaller fraction of the ingested ascorbic acid may do so either because he has been living on a diet containing an insufficient quantity of the vitamin, such that his tissues are depleted, or because some biochemical abnormality of his body operates to remove ascorbate from the blood serum very rapidly, perhaps by converting it rapidly into other substances. It was reported by VanderKamp in 1966 that patients with longstanding chronic schizophrenia required a loading dose of ascorbic acid about ten times greater than that required by other persons to cause the appearance of a certain amount in the urine, and this observation was verified by Herjanic and Moss-Herjanic (1967). The results of another loading test are shown in Figure 3 (Pauling and others; Chapter 2 in Hawkins and Pauling, 1973). In this study forty-four patients recently hospitalized with acute schizophrenia and forty-four other subjects were given 1.76 g of ascorbic acid by mouth and the fraction excreted in the urine in six hours was measured. There was a twenty-fold individual variation in this fraction, from 2 percent to 40 percent, with the schizophrenic patients excreting only about 60 percent as much as the others. This variation is probably partly nutritional and partly genetic in origin. The distribution functions suggest that there are three kinds of human beings with respect to their handling of ascorbic acid, the low excretors, the medium excretors, and the high excretors. This idea has not, however, been thoroughly tested as yet.

Some of the subjects in this study were given 1.76 g of ascorbic acid every day for eight days, and the fraction excreted in the six hours after the last dose was determined. Of sixteen low excretors (less than 17 percent excreted), eight had moved out of the low-excretor class, whereas the excretion of the other eight remained low. This observation suggests that these persons have an abnormal way of handling their ingested vitamin C. They might require a much larger intake to be in good health.

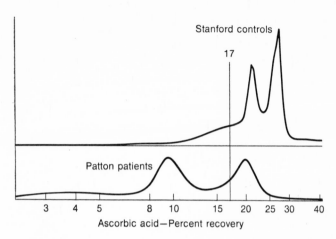

FIGURE 3

The upper curve shows the distribution function of Stanford students in respect to the fraction of a dose of ascorbic acid, taken by mouth, that is recovered in the urine in six hours. It is seen that many of the students eliminate about 25 percent of the ingested ascorbic acid in that period, a somewhat smaller group of students eliminate about 20 percent, and some of them eliminate a still smaller amount. The lower curve, for schizophrenic patients in Patton State Hospital, seems to show three similar groups, shifted somewhat to smaller amounts of ascorbic acid eliminated, and with a larger fraction of the patients eliminating only a small amount of the vitamin.

In Chapter 9 mention was made of several serious genetic diseases, such as phenylketonuria, galactosemia, and methylmalonicaciduria. Many of these diseases are now known, and some of them can be controlled by a large intake of an appropriate vitamin. It is harder to recognize a mild genetic disease than a serious one, but the mild genetic diseases may altogether cause more suffering than the serious ones, because so many more people suffer from them. It is likely than many of the low excretors of ascorbic acid shown in Figure 3 have a genetic defect such that a low intake of vitamin C is more damaging to them than to other people. For them a larger intake of the vitamin may be essential if they are to avoid a short and miserable life. At the present time it is very difficult to determine the nutritional needs of an individual person, except by trial of various intakes, but we may hope that reliable clinical tests that show the individual needs will be developed before long.

11

Side Effects of Vitamin C

When my book *Vitamin C and the Common Cold* was published in November 1970 it was greeted with strong criticism. Some of the criticism was directed at my failure to emphasize the possible danger of harmful long-term side effects resulting from the intake of several grams of vitamin C each day. This topic is treated in the following paragraphs.

VITAMIN C AS A LAXATIVE

One effect of vitamin C in large doses has been reported by many people. This is its effect as a laxative, its action in causing looseness of the bowels. For some people a single dose of 3 g taken on an empty stomach exerts too strong a laxative action, whereas the same amount taken at the end of a meal does not. One physician who treats patients with infectious diseases by having them take as much ascorbic acid as they can without discomfort has reported that most of them take between 15 g and 30 g per day (Cathcart, 1975). Virno et al. (1967) and Bietti (1967) have written that glaucoma patients taking 30 g to 40 g of ascorbic acid per day suffer from "diarrhea" for three or four days, but not thereafter.

Constipation can usually be controlled by adjusting the intake of vitamin C (Hoffer, 1971). To be in the best of health it may be wise to evacuate the contents of the lower bowel two or three times a day, rather than only once every day or every other day. To carry the waste matter around for a longer time than necessary might do some harm. On the other hand, moderately irritant laxatives, such as milk of magnesia, cascara sagrada, or sodium sulfate, might themselves cause some harm. Physicians often advise patients suffering from constipation to eat a good diet, including plenty of fruit and vegetables. This is good orthomolecular treatment, but the use of vitamin C, in addition to that in the fruit and vegetables, is also good orthomolecular treatment.

A large intake of vitamin C has also been reported to increase the production of intestinal gas (methane) in many people.

To minimize these effects, to the extent that they are undesirable, one might try various kinds of vitamin C and various ways of taking it (after meals, for example, as mentioned above). Some people say that they can handle the salt sodium ascorbate better than ascorbic acid, and for some a mixture of the two may be best.* Some undesirable effects might be attributable to the filter or binder or the coloring or

*Pure crystalline ascorbic acid, sodium ascorbate, and a 50:50 mixture of the two can be obtained retail from Bronson Pharmaceuticals, La Cañada, California, and some other sources.

flavoring additives in tablets, making it desirable to change the brand or to use the pure substances. For some people the timed-release tablets may solve the problem.

It should not surprise us that our intestinal tracts cause some temporary trouble for us when we ingest 5 g or 10 g of ascorbic acid per day, even though this quantity is indicated to be the optimum by the fact that animals manufacture this amount for themselves. The animals make it inside their bodies, in the liver or kidney. It does not pass into the stomach and intestines, except for the smaller amount obtained from their food. After we lost the ability to synthesize this nutrient and began eating foods that provided us with only a small amount, 1 g or 2 g per day, our digestive systems were not under any evolutionary pressure to adapt to the reception of larger amounts. We may have adapted to some extent to get along with smaller amounts, but there are indications, discussed elsewhere in this book, that our optimum intake is not less than the amount synthesized by other animals for their own benefit.

Some people have asked me if ascorbic acid, by acting as an acid, might not cause stomach ulcers. In fact, the gastric juice in the stomach contains a strong acid, and ascorbic acid, which is a weak acid, does not increase its acidity. Aspirin tablets and potassium chloride tablets can corrode the wall of the stomach and cause ulcers. Vitamin C keeps them from forming and helps to heal them (for references and additional discussion see Stone, 1972).

KIDNEY STONES

Eighteen days after the publication of my book *Vitamin C and the Common Cold,* a review of it appeared in *The Medical*

Letter, a nonprofit publication for physicians on drugs and therapeutics put out by Drug and Therapeutic Information, Inc., New York (*The Medical Letter,* 25 December 1970). This review was entirely unfavorable. It contained many strongly critical statements, most of which were false or misleading. These statements were then repeated in *The New York Times* (Altman, 1971) and many other newspapers, as well as in *Consumer Reports* (see the following chapter) and other magazines. I wrote a letter discussing the false and misleading statements, and asked *The Medical Letter* to publish it. This was not done; instead, on 28 May 1971 *The Medical Letter* published a second article on the subject, with the title "Vitamin C—Were the Trials Well Controlled and Are Large Doses Safe?", in which some of the earlier statements and the recommendation against the use of ascorbic acid were repeated.

One point raised by *The Medical Letter* is that vitamin C might have the adverse effect of causing kidney stones to form. The editors of this publication wrote that, "When 4 to 12 grams of vitamin C are taken daily for acidification of the urine, however, as in the management of some chronic urinary tract infections, precipitation of urate and cystine stones in the urinary tract can occur. Very large doses of vitamin C, therefore, should be avoided in patients with a tendency to gout, to formation of urate stones, or to cystinuria."

This statement is wrong. The editors might quite properly have written that very large doses of ascorbic acid should be avoided in these patients, but there is no reason for the patients to refrain from taking vitamin C in large doses, because it can be taken as sodium ascorbate, which does not acidify the urine. The statement made in *The Medical Letter* shows that the editors of the publication simply did not understand what they were writing about.

It is well known that there are two classes of kidney stones, and that a tendency to form them should be controlled in two quite different ways. The stones of one class, comprising nearly one half of all urinary calculi, are composed of calcium phosphate, magnesium ammonium phosphate, calcium carbonate, or mixtures of these substances. They tend to form in alkaline urine, and persons with a tendency to form them are advised to keep their urine acidic. A good way, probably the best way, to acidify the urine is to take 1 g or more of ascorbic acid each day. Ascorbic acid is used by many physicians for this purpose and for preventing infections of the urinary tract, especially infection by organisms that hydrolyze urea to form ammonia and in this way alkalize the urine and promote the formation of kidney stones of this class.

The kidney stones of the other class, which tend to form in acidic urine, are composed of calcium oxalate, uric acid, or cystine. Persons with a tendency to form these stones are advised to keep their urine alkaline. This can be achieved by their taking their vitamin C as sodium ascorbate or by taking ascorbic acid with just enough sodium hydrogen carbonate (ordinary baking soda) or other alkalizer to neutralize it.

Not a single case has been reported in the medical literature of a person who formed kidney stones because of a large intake of vitamin C. There is the possibility, however, that some people might have an increased tendency to form calcium oxalate kidney stones while taking a large amount of vitamin C. It is known that ascorbic acid can be oxidized to oxalic acid in the body. Lamden and Chrystowski (1954) studied fifty-one healthy male subjects with an ordinary intake of vitamin C (only that in their food), and found the average amount of oxalic acid excreted in the urine to be 38 mg (range 16 mg to 64 mg). The average increased by only 3 mg for 2 g per day additional ascorbic acid and by only 12 mg per day for 4 g. Additional intake of 8 g per day increased the excretion of oxalic acid by 45 mg, and of 9 g by 68 mg (average—as much as 150 mg was excreted by one subject). It seems likely that most people would not have trouble with oxalic acid while taking large doses of vitamin C, but a few might have to be careful, just as they have to refrain from eating spinach and rhubarb, which have a high oxalate content. A few people have a rare genetic disease that leads to the increased production of oxalic acid in their own cells (largely from the amino acid glycine), and one young man is known who converts about 15 percent of ingested ascorbic acid into oxalic acid, fifty times more than is converted by other people (Briggs, Garcia-Webb, and Davies, 1973). This man, and others who have the same genetic defect, must limit their intake of vitamin C.

VITAMIN C AND VITAMIN B_{12}

During the last two and a half years I have received many letters from people who were troubled by a report that large doses of vitamin C taken with food destroyed the vitamin B_{12} in the food, leading to a deficiency disease resembling pernicious anemia. I replied that the report was not reliable, because the conditions under which the food had been investigated in the laboratory were not closely similar to those for food that is swallowed and kept in the stomach. It has now been shown that the original report, by Herbert and Jacob (1974), was wrong, because of their use of an unreliable method of analysis, and that in fact vitamin C does not destroy the vitamin B_{12} in food to any significant extent.

Herbert and Jacob studied a meal with modest vitamin B_{12} content and a meal with high B_{12} content, the latter containing 90 g of grilled beef liver, which is known to be rich in B_{12}. Some of the meals had 100 mg, 250 mg, or 500 mg of ascorbic acid added. The meals were homogenized in a blender, held for 30 minutes at body temperature (37° C), and then analyzed for vitamin B_{12} by a radioactive-isotope method. The investigators reported that 500 mg of ascorbic acid added to the meal destroyed 95 percent of the vitamin B_{12} in the modest-B_{12} meal and nearly 50 percent in the high-B_{12} meal. They concluded that "High doses of vitamin C, popularly used as a home remedy against the common cold, destroy substantial amounts of vitamin B_{12} when ingested with foods. . . . Daily ingestion of 500 mg or more of ascorbic acid without regular evaluation of vitamin B_{12} status is probably unwise." This statement has been repeated in many articles on nutrition and health in newspapers and magazines during the last two and a half years.

It is known that pure hydroxycobalamin and pure cyano-cobalamin (forms of vitamin B_{12}) are attacked and destroyed (cyanocobalamin less rapidly) by ascorbic acid in the presence of oxygen and copper ions, but the amount of destruction reported by Herbert and Jacobs was surprisingly high. Moreover, there was evidence in the account of their results given by Herbert and Jacobs that something was wrong in their work. The amount of vitamin B_{12} reported by them from their analysis of the meals (without added ascorbic acid) was only about one eighth of that known to be present in the foods comprising the meals. It is known that some of the vitamin B_{12} in foods is tightly bound to proteins and other constituents of the foods. Biochemists developed some special procedures to release the bound vitamin. If these procedures are not used, only the amount of loosely bound B_{12} is determined in the analysis. Investigators in two different laboratories then repeated the work, using reliable analytical methods (Newmark, Scheiner, Marcus, and Prabhudesai, 1976). They found amounts of B_{12} in the two meals equal, to within 5 percent, to the amounts calculated from the food tables. Their amounts were six to eight times those reported by Herbert and Jacob, and, moreover, they found that addition of 100 mg, 250 mg, or 500 mg of ascorbic acid led to no change in the amount of B_{12} in the meal.

We may conclude from this work that the hazard ascribed to the intake with meals of moderately large amounts of vitamin C, 500 mg or more, by Herbert and Jacob does not exist. They were led to draw an incorrect conclusion by having used a poor method of chemical analysis for vitamin B_{12}.

EFFECT OF VITAMIN C ON CLINICAL TESTS

One of the reasons proposed by *Medical Letter* for not taking an increased amount of vitamin C is that the presence of vitamin C in the urine might cause the ordinary tests for glucose in the urine, a sign of diabetes, to give a false positive result. This fact is hardly an argument against taking the valuable substance vitamin C. It is instead an argument for developing reliable tests for glucose in the urine.

Brandt, Guyer, and Banks (1974) have shown how the tests for glucose in the urine can be modified to prevent interference by ascorbic acid. An even simpler way is to refrain from taking vitamin C on the day when the urine sample is obtained.

Another common test that is interfered with by ascorbic acid is that for blood in the stool, an indication of internal bleeding (Jaffe et al., 1975). Dr. Russell M. Jaffe of the National Institutes of Health, who discovered this effect, is now developing a more reliable test.

THE REBOUND EFFECT WITH VITAMIN C

When a person ingests an ordinary quantity of vitamin C each day the concentration of ascorbate in his blood remains constant at about 15 mg per liter. Spero and Anderson (1973) studied twenty-nine subjects who were put on an intake of 1 g, 2 g, or 4 g per day. Their blood levels rose at first to over 20 mg per liter, but after some days decreased. A similar effect was also noticed by Harris, Robinson, and Pauling (1973), and was attributed by them to increased metabolic utilization of the vitamin C in response to the increase in intake.

This phenomenon is well known in bacteria. The ordinary intestinal bacterium *E. coli* usually uses the simple sugar glucose as its source of carbon. It can also live on the disaccharide lactose (milk sugar). When a culture of *E. coli* is transferred from glucose to lactose it grows very slowly for a while, and then rapidly. In order to live on lactose the organism must contain an enzyme that splits lactose into two halves. *E. coli* is able to manufacture this enzyme, betagalactosidase, because it has the corresponding gene in its genetic material, but when it is living on glucose each cell in the culture contains only a dozen molecules of it. When it is transferred to a medium containing lactose each cell synthesizes several thousand molecules of the enzyme, permitting it to use the lactose more effectively.

This is called induced enzyme formation. It was discovered in 1900, and was carefully investigated by the French biologist Jacques Monod (b. 1910, d. 1976; received a Nobel Prize in Medicine, shared with François Jacob and André Lwoff, in 1965). Monod and his associates demonstrated that the rate of manufacture of the enzyme under the control of its specific gene is itself controlled by another gene, called a regulatory gene. When there is little or no lactose in the medium, the regulatory gene stops the synthesis of the enzyme. This decreases the unnecessary burden on the bacterium of man- ufacturing a useless enzyme. When lactose is present the regulatory gene starts the process of synthesizing the enzyme, in order that the lactose can be used as food.

The evidence indicates that human beings have similar regulatory genes that control the synthesis of the enzymes involved in the conversion of ascorbic acid into other sub- stances. These other substances, oxidation products, are valu- able; it is known, for example, that they are more effective in the control of cancer in animals than is ascorbic acid (Omura et al., 1974 and 1975). But ascorbic acid itself is also an important substance, directly involved in the synthesis of collagen and in other reactions in the human body. It would be catastrophic if the enzymes were to operate so efficiently as to convert all of the ascorbic acid and dehydroascorbic acid into oxidation products that do not have the same biochemical properties as the vitamin. For this reason the regulatory genes stop or slow down the manufacture of the enzymes when the intake of vitamin C is small. When the intake is large the enzymes are produced in larger amounts, permitting more of the ascorbic acid to be converted into the other useful substances.

When a person has been receiving a high intake of vitamin C for a few days or longer the amount of these enzymes is so large that if he stops the high intake, reverting to a low intake, most of the ascorbic acid in his blood is rapidly converted into other substances, and the concentration of ascorbic acid and dehydroascorbic acid in his blood becomes abnormally low. His resistance to disease may be decreased. This is the rebound effect.

The rebound effect lasts for a week or two (Spero and Toulin, 1974). By that time the amount of the enzymes has decreased to the normal value for a low intake, and the concentration of ascorbic acid in the blood has risen to its normal value. It is accordingly wise for people who have been taking a large amount of vitamin C and who decide to revert to a small intake to decrease the intake gradually, over a week or two, rather than suddenly.

The rebound effect probably is not very important for most people. Anderson, Suranyi, and Beaton (1974) checked the amount of winter illness (mainly colds) in their subjects during the month just after they had stopped taking their tablets of ascorbic acid or placebo. During this month the subjects who had been receiving 1 g or 2 g of vitamin C each day and those who had been receiving the placebo had nearly the same number of episodes of illness per person, 0.304 and 0.309, respectively. The mean values of number of days indoors per person, 0.384 and 0.409, and number of days off work, 0.221

and 0.268, were a little smaller for the first group than for the second, rather than the reverse, which would be expected if the rebound effect were important. Also, there was no greater amount of illness during the first half than the second half of the month.

Some people might suffer from an abnormality involving these regulatory genes. The presence of an excess of the enzymes that catalyze the oxidation of vitamin C might be responsible for the abnormality in metabolizing the vitamin that is observed for some schizophrenic subjects. The scare stories that have been published about rebound scurvy seem, however, to have no sound basis.

VITAMIN C AND PREGNANCY

It has been known for over thirty years that pregnant women need more vitamin C than other women. Part of the reason for this extra need is that the developing fetus needs a good supply of this vitamin, and there is a mechanism in the placenta for pumping vitamin C from the blood of the mother into that of the fetus. In one early study (Javert and Stander, 1943) the ascorbate concentration in the blood of the umbilical cord was found to be 14.3 mg per liter, four times that of the blood of the mother. Depletion of the maternal blood for the benefit of the infant continues even after parturition, as ascorbate is secreted in the mother's milk. Cow's milk is much less rich in vitamin C than human milk; the calf does not need extra vitamin C, because it manufactures its own in the cells of its liver.

In normal pregnancy women with the usual low intake of vitamin C have been reported to show a steady decrease in blood plasm concentration from 11 mg per liter (average for 246 women) to 5 mg per liter at 4 months and then to 3.5 mg at full term (Javert and Stander, 1943). These low values correspond to poor health, not only for the mother but also for the infant. A low value of the blood concentration of vitamin C has been shown to be correlated with incidence of hemorrhagic disease of the newborn. Javert and Stander concluded that for good health an intake of 200 mg per day is needed by the pregnant woman, and it is likely that for most pregnant women the optimum intake is still greater, 1 g or more per day. Other nutritional needs must, of course, also be satisfied. Brewer (1966) has emphasized that a good intake of protein and other nutrients is essential to prevent puerperal eclampsia and that the diuretics and diet restrictions that are used to control the increase in weight during pregnancy are harmful.

A good intake of vitamin C has great value in controlling threatened, spontaneous, and habitual abortion. In their study of seventy-nine women with threatened, previous spontaneous, or habitual abortion Javert and Stander (1943) had 91-percent success with thirty-three patients who received vitamin C, together with bioflavonoids and vitamin K (only three abortions), whereas all of the forty-six patients who did not receive the vitamin aborted. In his analysis of the management of habitual abortion Greenblatt (1955) concluded that vitamin C with bioflavonoids and vitamin K is the best treatment, the next best thing progesterone, vitamin E, and thyroid extract.

During the last seven years various authorities in the field of nutrition who write newspaper columns have repeatedly stated that a high intake of vitamin C can cause abortions. The basis for this statement seems to be a brief paper by two physicians in the Soviet Union, Samborskaya and Ferdman (1966). They reported that twenty women in the age range twenty to forty years whose menstruation was delayed by ten to fifteen days were given 6 g of ascorbic acid by mouth on each of three successive days, and that sixteen of them then menstruated. I wrote to Samborskaya and Ferdman, asking if any test of pregnancy had been carried out. In reply they sent me only another copy of their paper.

Hoffer (1971) has stated that he has used megadoses of ascorbic acid, 3 g to 30 g per day, with over a thousand patients since 1953, and has not seen one case of kidney-stone formation, miscarriage, excessive dehydration, or any other serious toxicity.

It seems unlikely that ascorbic acid causes abortions to any great extent, although it may help to control difficulties with menstruation. Lahann (1970) has reviewed the literature, especially that in German and Austrian journals. He concluded that noticeable improvement in menstruation had been observed through the oral intake of 200 mg to 1,000 mg of ascorbic acid per day. Moreover, the utilization of ascorbic acid increases sharply in the course of the menstrual cycle, especially at the time of ovulation, and measurement of this utilization can be used for determining the end of ovulation and accordingly for determining the time of optimum conception in relation to the problem of overcoming sterility (Paeschke and Vasterling, 1968).

12

The Medical Establishment
and Vitamin C

In the Introduction, I mentioned that whereas many people believe that vitamin C helps prevent colds, most physicians deny that this vitamin has much value. My experiences since the publication of my book *Vitamin C and the Common Cold* (in December 1970) have substantiated this idea, and have stimulated me to attempt to explain the fact.

Many physicians have written me that they find ascorbic acid to be effective in controlling the common cold and other infections of the respiratory tract, and use it in treating themselves, members of their families, and patients. (Some hundreds of nonphysicians also have written me about their successful use of ascorbic acid, usually over a period of years.) I have received only three or four letters from physicians who are convinced that vitamin C has no such effectiveness. It is likely, however, that this small number is misleading—the skeptics do not write to me.

Cortez F. Enloe, Jr., M.D., editor of *Nutrition Today,* in an editorial article (1971) on my book, mentioned that he had not found one physician among his friends or among those attending a meeting of a state medical society who "would admit to having even read the book." I surmise that most physicians have read neither this book nor any of the articles describing the controlled studies that have been made of ascorbic acid in relation to the common cold. I estimate that one American physician in a thousand has read the 1942 article by Cowan, Diehl, and Baker, and that one in ten thousand has read the 1961 article by Ritzel. The opinions of all but a handful are secondhand.

Almost all physicians rely upon the statements made by authorities. This situation is inevitable. The practicing physician is too busy to make a thorough study of the complex and often voluminous original literature on every medical topic. For example, a physician in Albuquerque, New Mexico, wrote a letter to the local newspaper, saying that it had been shown that vitamin C has no value at all in protecting against the common cold and other respiratory diseases. I wrote to him, asking him which published accounts of investigations he had based his statement upon. He replied that he was a gynecologist, and knew little about infectious diseases; he had based his statement in the newspaper on information that had been given to him by his old professor, Dr. F. J. Stare, by telephone. The physician had relied upon an authority who, like many members of the medical establishment, has ignored the mounting evidence in favor of the treatment of the common cold with vitamin C.

THE MEDICAL INVESTIGATORS

Some of the medical investigators themselves have failed to analyze their own observations in a sound way and to act in accordance with these results. Cowan, Diehl, and Baker (1942) provide an example. These three physicians carried out a careful study of ascorbic acid (about 200 mg per day), in comparison with a placebo, with 363 subjects over a period of twenty-eight weeks. They observed a decreased incidence of colds for the ascorbic-acid group (relative to the placebo group) by 15 percent and a decreased severity by 19 percent (Chapter 6). These decreases are statistically significant; according to the rules generally accepted by statisticians, they should not be ignored. Nevertheless, Cowan, Diehl, and Baker did ignore the results. In the summary of their paper, which is the only part that would be read by most readers of the *Journal of the American Medical Association*, they omitted mention of these facts. Their summary consists of a single sentence, as follows: "This controlled study yields no indication that either large doses of vitamin C or large doses of vitamins A, B_1, B_2, C, D, and nicotinic acid have any important effect on the number or severity of infections of the upper respiratory tract when administered to young adults who presumably are already on a reasonably adequate diet."

In my opinion this statement is incorrect. The vitamin-C subjects had only 69 percent as much illness with the common cold (as measured by days of illness per subject, the product of the number of colds per subject and the days of illness per cold) as the placebo subjects. This surely is an important effect, the result of a 15 percent decrease in incidence and a 19 percent decrease in severity. The only explanation of the action of

Cowan, Diehl, and Baker in writing the summary in this way is that they did not consider the observed effect important; but surely most people would consider it important to be able to cut their amount of illness with the common cold by nearly one third. A letter by Dr. Diehl in *The New York Times* (1970) indicates that he still thought that Cowan, Diehl, and Baker did not obtain positive results. In my reply (1971d) I pointed out that Dr. Diehl and I agreed about the facts but disagreed about the word "important," and that Cowan, Diehl, and Baker had made an error of judgment in omitting from their summary mention of the *fact* that they had observed a statistically significant protective effect of ascorbic acid against the common cold.

Glazebrook and Thomson (1942) also misconstrued their own observations in the summary of their paper. It is mentioned in Chapter 6 that in their main study, with 435 subjects, they found the incidence of colds and tonsillitis in the ascorbic-acid group to be 13 percent less than for the controls. The incidence of colds alone was 17 percent less in this main study and 12 percent less in a second study, with 150 subjects (incidence of colds and tonsillitis 25 percent less). These facts, presented in the body of the paper, are not repeated in the summary. Instead, the statement is made, contrary to the facts, that "the incidences of common cold and tonsillitis were the same in the two groups."

Similar failure to present in the summaries of their papers a correct account of the results of their work can be found also in the reports of other investigators.

The actions of these investigators in understating their observations in the summaries of their papers may have been the result of a sort of conservatism and restraint, the feeling that one should not claim that a therapeutic or preventive effect has been observed unless it is a large and obvious one. It is my opinion that feelings of this sort, admirable though they may be, do not justify an incorrect description of one's observations. One must always strive for accuracy. It is just as wrong to understate one's findings as to overstate them. There is no doubt that the original investigators themselves have been partly responsible for the failure of the medical establishment to recognize the significance of the observations.

THE ATTITUDE OF THE MEDICAL AUTHORITIES

The attitude of the medical authorities in recent years is illustrated by the statement in the editorial article in *Nutrition Reviews* (1967), quoted in the Introduction of this book, that there is no conclusive evidence that ascorbic acid has any protective or therapeutic effect on the course of the common cold in healthy people. The study of the evidence made by the anonymous author of this editorial article was clearly a careless and superficial one, in that, as is mentioned in Chapter 6, he erroneously reported that Ritzel (1961) had observed only a 39 percent reduction in the number of days of illness and a 36 percent reduction in the incidence of symptoms, the correct values being nearly twice as great (61 percent and 65 percent, respectively). There is no indication in the editorial article that the author made any attempt to analyze the evidence in the published papers, to find out whether the statement could be made that the evidence shows with statistical significance that ascorbic acid either has a protective or therapeutic effect or does not have such an effect (of a given assumed magnitude). It seems not unlikely that the author was misled by the incorrect summary statements of some investigators, as mentioned above, and by the prevailing medical opinion, and that this bias led to the superficiality of his study.

Even after the first publication of my book *Vitamin C and the Common Cold,* on 7 December 1970, when the evidence was clearly brought to the attention of the medical authorities, they continued to deny the existence of the evidence. This denial of the existence of the evidence was sometimes accompanied by statements that contradict or misconstrue the facts.

Among the authorities who denied the existence of this evidence was Dr. Charles C. Edwards, the chief of the United States Food and Drug Administration. On 29 December 1970 he told reporters that the run on drugstores for vitamin C since publication of my book was "ridiculous," and stated that "there is no scientific evidence and never have been any meaningful studies indicating that vitamin C is capable of preventing or curing colds" (United Press International dispatch by Craig A. Palmer, 29 December 1971, printed in many newspapers). I wrote several letters to Commissioner Edwards, asking him to explain how he could reconcile this statement with the existence of the evidence summarized in my book, especially the results obtained by Ritzel. In his replies, which included material by Allan L. Forbes, M.D., Deputy Director of the Division of Nutrition of the Food and Drug Administration, several critical comments were made about the work of Ritzel and of other investigators quoted in my book. It was concluded, however, that Ritzel "does present what seem to be meaningful data." Nevertheless, the official opinion about vitamin C and the common cold remained unchanged.

On 18 December 1970 Commissioner Edwards telephoned me and asked me to come to Washington for a conference about this matter with the Food and Drug Administration. I agreed, and suggested that some questions be clarified by correspondence before the meeting. This clarification by correspondence was carried out, as described in the preceding paragraph, and in June 1971 I wrote Commissioner Edwards that I would come immediately to Washington for the conference, at a date convenient to him. He then withdrew the invitation, and the conference has never taken place.

Despite the repeated findings that an increased intake of vitamin C provides some protection against respiratory illnesses and other diseases, as summarized in Chapter 6 and elsewhere in this book, our Federal health agencies continue to deny that it has any value. For example, in August 1975 the National Institutes of Health issued a pamphlet (566-AMDD-975-B) containing many incorrect statements: "the body uses only the amount of ascorbic acid it needs and excretes the rest in the urine"; "other questions about the safety of high doses of ascorbic acid include its possible affect [sic] on fertility and the fetus, interference with the treatment of patients whose urine must be kept alkaline . . ."; "recent reports further demonstrate that high doses of vitamin C destroy substantial amounts of the vitamin B_{12} in food." It is stated in the pamphlet that it is reasonable to assume that 45 mg per day is sufficient to prevent disease and maintain health. The only mention of the evidence is the assertion that the studies are unconvincing.

The authors of the authoritative reference books and textbooks have failed to assess the evidence about vitamin C in a proper way. For example, in the sixth edition of the book *Human Nutrition and Dietetics* by Davidson, Passmore, Brock,

and Truswell, published in 1975, there is the following statement on page 163:

> The claim by Pauling (1970) that the consumption of 1 or 2 g
> per day promotes optimum health and protects against the
> common cold rests on slender evidence. In clinical trials large
> doses of the vitamin given to students in America and in Scot-
> land (Cowan et al., 1942; Glazebrook and Thomson, 1942)
> provided no unequivocal protection against colds. At the
> Common Cold Research Unit in Salisbury a dose of 3 g per
> day of ascorbic acid did not reduce the number of infections
> produced by inoculating volunteers with viruses causing upper
> respiratory infections (Walker et al., 1967).

In fact, in the two 1942 studies there was a statistically
significant amount of protection, 30 to 50 percent decreased
amount of illness, even though the daily intake of ascorbic acid
was quite small, only 200 mg. Davidson and his coauthors do
not mention the work by Ritzel, with 1,000 mg per day and 67
percent protection, or the several other studies mentioned in
Chapter 6 and Appendix III of this book. They knew about
Ritzel's study, because one of the authors, Passmore, wrote a
review of my book *Vitamin C and the Common Cold,* in which
Ritzel's work is discussed (Passmore, 1971). Why these authorities in the field of nutrition should misinterpret and
ignore the evidence is not clear.

Their statement that Walker et al. showed that a dose of 3 g
per day did not reduce the number of infections in volunteers
inoculated with cold viruses is also not quite true. In this study
the vitamin-C subjects had 6 percent fewer colds than the
placebo subjects, and their colds were 9 percent less severe.
Moreover, the design of the study had a serious flaw, in that the
administration of the vitamin was stopped shortly after the
onset of the colds (see Appendix III).

THE MEDICAL LETTER

It is mentioned in the preceding chapter that *The Medical Letter,* a publication on drugs and therapeutics for physicians, published an unfavorable review of my book *Vitamin C and the Common Cold* on 25 December 1970. I wrote a letter discussing the false and misleading statements in their review, and asked *The Medical Letter* to publish it. This was not done; instead, on 28 May 1971 *The Medical Letter* published a second article on the subject, with the title "Vitamin C—Were the Trials Well Controlled and Are Large Doses Safe?," in which some of the earlier statements and the recommendation against the use of ascorbic acid were repeated.

In the first article in *The Medical Letter* it was said that I had relied on uncontrolled studies. The statement was made that ". . . a controlled trial of the effectiveness of vitamin C against upper respiratory infections must be conducted over a long period and include many hundreds of persons to give meaningful results. No such trial has been performed."

This statement is false, as could have been ascertained by the writer of the article simply by reading my book. The study by Cowan, Diehl, and Baker, for example, was a controlled study that showed a statistically significant protective effect of ascorbic acid in comparison with a placebo; it was conducted over a long period (twenty-eight weeks) and included hundreds of persons (363). In the second article, *The Medical Letter* gives as reasons for rejecting the results of the study by Cowan, Diehl, and Baker that the study was not double-blind (although Dr. Cowan himself says that it was) and that allocation of subjects to the ascorbic-acid group and the placebo group was not randomized (although the investigators describe their method of randomization in their paper).

The Medical Letter also discussed the study by Ritzel in its second article, raising some rather trivial points of criticism, such as that Ritzel had not given the ages and sex of the subjects. His paper indicated that the subjects were all school-boys, and in a letter to me Ritzel verified that they were all boys, and said that they were fifteen to seventeen years old. *The Medical Letter* also raised the question of the possible formation of kidney stones, as mentioned in Chapter 11. The weakness of the arguments advanced by *The Medical Letter* and some other critics caused a Canadian physician, Dr. A. Hoffer, to make the following comment (1971): "[These critics] use two sets of logic. Before they are prepared to look at Dr. Pauling's hypothesis, they demand proof of the most rigorous kind. But when arguing against his views, they refer to evidence of the flimsiest sort for the toxicity of ascorbic acid."

Popular writers are, of course, misled by such authoritative misstatements. In a thoroughly unreliable article in *Reader's Digest* (Ross, 1971), there is the sentence, "But some of these patients [who had taken 4,000 to 10,000 mg of vitamin C a day] have developed kidney stones." My request to *Reader's Digest* and the author of the article to give me the references to the medical literature about these patients was unsuccessful. *The Medical Letter* did not mention any patients in whom ascorbic acid had caused kidney stones to form, but mentioned only such a possibility.

CONSUMER REPORTS

Consumer Reports is a publication, now in its fortieth year, that purports "to provide consumers with information and counsel on consumer goods and services, to give information on all matters relating to the expenditure of the family income, and to initiate and to cooperate with individual and group efforts seeking to create and maintain decent living standards." It is published by a nonprofit organization, Consumers Union, established in 1936. My wife and I subscribed to *Consumer Reports* when it began, and over a period of thirty-five years we placed some confidence in its recommendations, as have many of its other subscribers, who now number in the millions.

The usual procedure of Consumers Union is to purchase products on the open market, to carry out "laboratory tests, controlled-use tests and/or expert judgments of the purchased samples," and to assign ratings on this basis. The organization pledges that "any opinions entering into its Ratings shall be as free of bias as it is possible to make them."

For example, in preparing a three-page report on disposable diapers (*Consumer Reports,* February 1971, pages 81 to 83), the organization purchased supplies of ten brands of diapers, examined their construction carefully, had comparative use tests carried out by twenty-five mothers, and then rated the diapers.

In the same issue of *Consumer Reports,* pages 113 and 114, in the section on Health and Medicine, there is a report entitled "Vitamin C, Linus Pauling and the Common Cold." It is a thoroughly biased report, consisting almost entirely of false statements and seriously misleading statements.

In its report, Consumers Union does not describe any tests that it carried out to determine the value of vitamin C in decreasing the incidence and severity of the common cold. Consumers Union could have rendered a real service to its members and other readers of *Consumer Reports* by purchasing vitamin C and some placebo tablets and carrying out a double-blind study, with its employees and members of their families as subjects. The number of employees, the normal incidence of colds, and the effectiveness of vitamin C when used as described in this book are such that results with statistical significance could have been obtained during the period January to April 1971. These results, either supporting the statements or not supporting them, could then have been published in the issue of *Consumer Reports* for June 1971. These actions would have constituted a real service to consumers, of the sort that Consumers Union claims to provide.

Instead, Consumers Union was guilty of a serious disservice to its supporters, in that it rushed into print an intemperate and completely unreliable account of my book, ending with an allegation of social irresponsibility: "Whatever the merits of increasing vitamin C allowances (and they should be explored), a socially responsible approach would dictate that toxicity studies should precede any efforts to encourage people to take large amounts of any vitamin."

The article contained ten false or seriously misleading statements, some of which were the same as those made by *The Medical Letter* discussed above. I immediately (10 February 1971) asked that a statement of correction, retraction, and apology be published in *Consumer Reports*. I received an answer, stating that the matter was being carefully considered. My wife and I then met with the president and another member of the board of directors. The president said that the organization was not planning to publish a statement about the article. I then asked if *Consumer Reports* would publish a discussion of the article by a distinguished pharmacologist who was interested in the matter but had not taken a position about it. The president said that this possibility would be considered. It was later rejected by *Consumer Reports*.

This consumers' organization, Consumers Union, published an article containing false and misleading statements about a matter of importance to nearly every consumer, and then refused to publish a correction.

After five years, *Consumers Reports* has published another article (February 1976), with the title "Is Vitamin C Really Good for Colds?" In this article reference is made to four of the controlled trials that have been carried out, but some of the best ones, such as that of Ritzel and that of Coulehan and his collaborators (Chapter 6), are not mentioned. The conclusion is reached that a daily intake of 120 mg can be recommended. Some of the old ideas that are now known to be false are repeated, such as the belief that higher amounts than about 120 mg per day are simply excreted in the urine and are accordingly wasted. *Consumer Reports* has thus taken a small step in the right direction since 1971, but still has a long way to go.

THE AMERICAN MEDICAL ASSOCIATION

For many years the stand of the American Medical Association, as expressed especially by Dr. Philip L. White, its principal spokesman on nutrition and health, has been that vitamin C has no value in preventing or treating the common cold or other diseases (White, 1975). On 10 March 1975 the AMA issued a statement to the press with the heading "Vitamin C will not prevent or cure the common cold." The basis for this quite negative statement was said to be two papers published on that day in the *Journal of the American Medical Association* (Karlowski et al., 1975; Dykes and Meier, 1975). Karlowski

and his associates had made a study of ascorbic acid in relation
to the common cold, with employees of the National Institutes
of Health as the subjects. This study is discussed in Appendix
III, where it is pointed out that the amount of illness per person
was 20 percent less for the vitamin-C subjects than for the
placebo subjects. The difference was not zero, as was suggested
by the AMA press release. The paper by Dykes and Meier was
a review of some other studies. The results observed by Ritzel
(1961), Sabiston and Radomski (1974), and some other investigators were, however, not presented. Despite their incom-
plete coverage of the evidence, Dykes and Meier concluded
that the studies seemed to show that vitamin C decreases the
amount of illness with the common cold, although in their
opinion its protective effect might not be large enough to be
clinically important. Thus their review of the evidence did not
provide any basis for the AMA statement that vitamin C will
not prevent or cure the common cold.

In order to present to the readers of the *Journal of the
American Medical Association* (JAMA) an account of all of the
evidence, I at once prepared a thorough but brief analysis of
thirteen controlled trials and submitted it to the editor on 19
March. He returned it to me twice, with suggestions for minor
revisions, which I made. Finally, on 24 September, six months
after I had submitted the article to him, he wrote me that it was
not wholly convincing and that he had decided to reject the
article and not publish it in JAMA. It was later published in
Medical Tribune (Pauling, 1976b).

It is my opinion that it is quite improper for the editor of the
Journal of the American Medical Association (or of any other
journal) to follow the policy of publishing only those papers
that support only one side of a scientific or medical question,

and also to interfere with the proper discussion of the question by holding a paper that had been submitted to him for half a year, during which period, according to accepted custom, the paper could not be submitted to another journal. This is not the only example of this sort of action by the editor of JAMA. The paper by Herbert and Jacob in which the claim was made that vitamin C taken with a meal destroys the vitamin B_{12} in the food and may cause a serious disease similar to pernicious anemia was published in JAMA (Chapter 11). When Newmark and his co-workers found that the claim could not be substantiated, and that in fact vitamin C does not destroy the vitamin B_{12} in the food, they sent their paper to the editor of JAMA, which seems clearly to be the place where the correction should be published. He held it for half a year, and then refused to publish it, thus delaying its publication in another journal and preventing many of the readers of the original article by Herbert and Jacobs from learning that their results were incorrect. These actions suggest that the American Medical Association works to protect American physicians from information that runs counter to its own prejudices. The evidence indicates that the AMA is prejudiced against vitamin C.

MODERN MEDICINE

The editor of JAMA and his advisors have a hard task to handle. Medicine is an extremely complicated subject. It is to a large extent based on sciences—physics, physical chemistry, organic chemistry, biochemistry, molecular biology, bacteriology, virology, genetics, pharmacology, and others—but it has not yet become a science. No one can know thoroughly more than a small part of medicine. Moreover, many physicians are limited in their scientific knowledge and have not had any experience in the field of scientific discovery. They do not know how to greet and how to assess new ideas.

The literature of science and medicine has now become so extensive that an editor may form his opinions on the basis of only a small part of the existing evidence. The editor of JAMA may have been too busy to look thoroughly into the vitamin-C question. The distinguished editor of *Modern Medicine*, Dr. Irvine H. Page, was on unsure ground when he wrote the editorial "Are truth and plain dealing going out of style? When even responsible investigators use shady tactics to promote their 'discoveries', it's no wonder that the public loses confidence in the scientific establishment," published in the 15 January 1976 issue of *Modern Medicine.* Several references to me that seem to have been based on profound misunderstandings were made. These were all corrected by Dr. Page in the 1 July 1976 issue of *Modern Medicine.* For instance, in his 15 January editorial he had written "To me, the most tragic example of self-deception was that in which Dr. Linus Pauling—twice a Nobel prizewinner—proposed and exploited the use of huge doses of vitamin C for the common cold." In his 1 July retraction he wrote "I withdraw this statement and regret the unjustified use of the pejorative words 'self-deception' and 'exploited' in connection with Dr. Pauling. . . . I regret that because of a misunderstanding I improperly claimed that Dr. Pauling demanded that his critics prove him wrong. Dr. Pauling in fact presented in his 1970 book *Vitamin C and the Common Cold* and in his articles a reasonable summary of the published reports of the several controlled studies that had been made, together with his own discussion and conclusions. He has not demanded that his critics prove him wrong, although he has urged them to examine the evidence. . . . The high opinion that this magazine has of Dr. Pauling is indicated by our action in giving him the Modern Medicine Award for Distinguished Achievement in 1963 for his discovery that sickle cell anemia is a molecular disease." Dr. Page also said that physicians should provide reliable information about such major public-health topics as nutrition (including the use of vitamin C), drugs, immunizations, and life styles, and by their own deportment earn and keep the respect and confidence of those they hope to benefit by preventive medicine. In addition, *Modern Medicine* published in the 1 July 1976 issue a paper by me on the case for vitamin C in maintaining health and preventing disease.

Modern Medicine seems to be developing a more open-minded attitude toward the recent progress in nutrition and preventive medicine, following the lead of another medical magazine, *Medical Tribune,* which over the years has continually been free from bias of this sort. I hope that in the course of time some improvement will become discernible in the publications of the American Medical Association.

Physicians must be conservative in the practice of medicine, but also the medical profession needs to be open to new ideas, if medicine is to progress. A new idea, that large amounts of vitamins might help in controlling disease, was discussed about forty years ago, but was not properly developed. Claus W. Jungeblut, the physician who first showed that ascorbic acid can inactivate viruses and provide some protection against viral diseases, became discouraged by the poor reception given his idea and went into another field of medicine. He advanced an interesting argument, new to me, in a letter to me on 10 February 1971: "I have read with great interest your recently published book *Vitamin C and the Common Cold* and wish to offer my congratulations for your efforts in bringing to the fore, and hopefully to practical solution, an age-old vexing medical problem. The chapter called 'Vitamin C and Evolution' seems to me particularly full of imaginative thinking. One might even go a step further here by asking why the *guinea pig*, of all common laboratory animals, shares with man certain physiological characteristics that include susceptibility not only to scurvy but also to anaphylactic shock, diphtheritic intoxication, pulmonary tuberculosis, a poliomyelitis-like neurotropic virus infection, and last but not least a form of viral leukemia that is indistinguishable from its human counterpart. None of the vitamin-C-synthesizing laboratory animals (rabbits, mice, rats, hamsters, etc.) answer positively to this call."

Dr. Jungeblut, who died in 1976, lived long enough to see the development of greatly increased activity in the field in which he carried on his pioneering work. There is no doubt that vitamin C has much value in controlling various diseases, but we shall not be sure how great its value is until more studies have been made.

13

Vitamin C and Drugs Compared

Ascorbic acid, vitamin C, is a food—an essential food, required by human beings for life and good health. It is safe, even when taken in very large amounts, far larger than the amounts that are needed to combat the common cold. Some people may find it desirable to take it together with some other food, in order that it not have a laxative action; this suggestion is essentially the only warning that need be made. There is no reason to fear that children will harm themselves with ascorbic acid. Its sour taste is likely to keep a child from eating very much, and he would not become seriously ill even if he were to eat several spoonfuls. Ascorbic acid is described in reference books as essentially nontoxic. Animals receiving daily amounts that correspond to 350 g (over three-quarters of a pound) per day for a man developed no symptoms of toxicity. With respect to safety, ascorbic acid is ideal.

The drugs that are used in tremendous amounts for treating the common cold, and that are advertised to an irritatingly great extent on television and radio and in newspapers and magazines, are much different; they are harmful and dangerous, and are themselves responsible for much illness and many deaths. They do not control the viral infection, but only the symptoms, to some extent, whereas vitamin C controls the infection itself, as well as the symptoms.

Aspirin is an example of a drug with low toxicity and few side effects. This drug, which is the chemical substance acetylsalicylic acid, is present in most cold medicines. The fatal dose for an adult is 20 g to 30 g. The ordinary aspirin tablet contains 324 mg (5 grains); hence 60 to 90 tablets can kill an adult, and a smaller amount can kill a child. Aspirin is the most common single poison used by suicides (it is second only to the group of substances used in sleeping pills). About 15 percent of accidental poisoning deaths of young children are caused by aspirin. Many lives would be saved if the medicine chest contained ascorbic acid in place of aspirin and the other cold medicines.

Some people show a severe sensitivity to aspirin, such that a decrease in circulation of the blood and difficulty in breathing follow the ingestion of 0.3 to 1 g (one to three tablets).

The symptoms of mild aspirin poisoning are burning pain in the mouth, throat, and abdomen, difficulty in breathing, lethargy, vomiting, ringing in the ears, and dizziness. More severe poisoning leads to delirium, fever, sweating, incoordination, coma, convulsions, cyanosis (blueness of the skin), failure of kidney function, respiratory failure, and death.

Aspirin, like other salicylates, has the property that in concentrated solution it can attack and dissolve tissues. An aspirin tablet in the stomach may attack the stomach wall and cause the development of a bleeding ulcer.

There are several other substances closely related to aspirin that have analgesic properties (the ability to decrease the sensitivity to pain) and antipyretic properties (the ability to lower increased body temperature) and are present in some of the popular cold medicines. One of these is salicylamide (the amide of salicylic acid). It has about the same toxicity as aspirin: 20 g to 30 g is the lethal dose for an adult.

The closely related analgesic substances acetanilide (N-phenylacetamide), phenacetin (acetophenetidin), and acetaminophen (p-hydroxyacetanilide) are used alone or in combination with other drugs in a number of cold medicines, in amounts of 150 mg to 200 mg per tablet. These substances damage the liver and kidneys. A single dose of 0.5 g to 5 g may cause fall of blood pressure, failure of kidney function, and death by respiratory failure.

Many of the cold medicines available without prescription contain not only aspirin or some other analgesic but also an anihistamine and an antitussive (to control severe coughing). For example, one preparation, recommended on the box for "Fast temporary relief of cold symptoms and accompanying coughs, sinus congestion, headache, the symptoms of hay fever," contains in each tablet 12 mg of the antihistamine methapyrilene hydrochloride and 5 mg of the antitussive dextromethorphan hydrobromide, as well as some phenacetin, salicylamide, and other substances. In the *Handbook of Poisoning* (Dreisbach, 1969) it is reported that the death of a small child was caused by the estimated amount 100 mg of methapyrilene (114 mg of the hydrochloride). At least twenty deaths of children have resulted from accidental poisoning by antihistamines. The estimated fatal dose for these reported poisonings lies in the range 10 mg to 50 mg per kilogram body weight for phenindamine, methapyrilene, diphenhydramine, and pyrilamine, and is probably about the same for many other antihistamines. These substances are more toxic than aspirin; one or two grams might cause the death of an adult.

These medicines often cause side effects, such as drowsiness and dizziness, even when taken in the recommended amounts. On the package there is usually a warning about the possibility of poisoning, for example,

> Keep this and all medicines out of children's reach. In case of accidental overdose, contact a physician immediately.

Moreover, there is often a more extensive warning, such as the following:

> CAUTION: Children under 12 should use only as directed by a physician. If symptoms persist or are unusually severe, see a physician. Do not exceed recommended dosage. Not for frequent or prolonged use. If excessive dryness of the mouth occurs, decrease dosage. Discontinue use if rapid pulse, dizziness, skin rash, or blurring of vision occurs. Do not drive or operate machinery as this preparation may cause drowsiness in some persons. Individuals with high blood pressure, heart disease, diabetes, thyroid disease, glaucoma or excessive pressure within the eye, and elderly persons (where undiagnosed glaucoma or excessive pressure within the eye may be present) should use only as directed by physician. Persons with undiagnosed glaucoma may experience eye pain; if this occurs discontinue use and see physician immediately.

The substance dextromethorphan hydrobromide, mentioned above as an antitussive, controls severe coughing by exerting a depressant effect on the brain. Also, the related substance codeine (as codeine phosphate) in amounts 15 mg to

60 mg every three or four hours is often prescribed by physicians for severe coughing. In most states of the United States codeine is not present in the medicines sold without prescription, but many of these medicines contain some other antitussive, such as dextromethorphan. The minimum fatal dose of these substances ranges from 100 mg to 1 g for an adult; much less for infants and more for narcotic addicts.

Some non-prescription cold medicines also contain belladonna alkaloids (atropine sulfate, hyoscyamine sulfate, scopolamine hydrobromide) in amounts as great as 0.2 mg per capsule. These drugs serve to dilate the bronchi and prevent spasms. They are intensely poisonous; the fatal dose in children may be as low as 10 mg. Side effects that may occur from ordinary doses are abnormal dryness of the mouth, blurred vision, slow beating of the heart, and retention of the urine.

Phenylpropanolamine hydrochloride (25 mg per tablet in some cold medicines) and phenylephrine hydrochloride (5 mg per tablet) serve to decrease nasal congestion and dilate the bronchi. These and related drugs, such as epinephrine and amphetamine, are also used in nose drops. It is estimated that one to ten percent of users of such nose drops have reactions from overdosage, such as chronic nasal congestion or personality changes with a psychic craving to continue the use of the drug. Fatalities are rare. The estimated fatal dose for children ranges from 10 mg for epinephrine to 200 mg for phenyl propanolamine.

The prescriptions of physicians for treating colds and other respiratory ailments contain these drugs and other drugs that are equally toxic or more toxic and have a similar incidence of side reactions.

Instead of the warning

> KEEP THIS MEDICINE OUT
> OF REACH OF CHILDREN!

carried by cold medicines, I think that they should say

> KEEP THIS MEDICINE OUT
> OF REACH OF EVERYBODY!
> USE ASCORBIC ACID INSTEAD!

The people of the United States spend about $500 million per year on cold medicines. These medicines do not prevent the colds. They may decrease somewhat the misery of the cold, but they also do harm, because of their toxicity and their side effects.

The natural, essential food ascorbic acid, taken in the right amounts at the right time, would prevent most of these colds from developing and would in most cases greatly decrease the intensity of the symptoms in those that do develop. Ascorbic acid is nontoxic, whereas all the cold drugs are toxic, and some of them cause severe side reactions in many people. In every respect, ascorbic acid is to be preferred to the dangerous and only partially effective analgesics, antipyretics, antihistamines, antitussives, bronchodilators, antispasmodics, and central-nervous-system depressants that constitute most medicines sold for relief of the common cold.

14

How to Control
the Common Cold
and the Flu

The following recommendations about intake of ascorbic acid are based upon the evidence and arguments presented in the earlier chapters of this book, including especially those in the publications of Stone and Régnier, as well as my own observations.

Williams and Deason have concluded that there is a twenty-fold range in the needs of individual guinea pigs for ascorbic acid, and that the range of needs of individual human beings is probably not smaller (Chapter 10). These recommendations include recognition of this biochemical individuality.

First, for good health I recommend the regular ingestion of an adequate amount of ascorbic acid. I estimate that for many people 1 g to 2 g per day (1,000 mg to 2,000 mg per day) is approximately the optimum rate of ingestion. There is evidence that some people remain in very good health, including freedom from the common cold, year after year through the ingestion of only 250 mg of ascorbic acid per day. The requirements of a few people for ascorbic acid may be expected to be even smaller. For some people optimum health may require larger amounts, up to 5 g per day or more.

The level of ascorbic acid in the blood reaches a maximum in two or three hours after the ingestion of a moderate quantity, and then gradually decreases, as the ascorbic acid is eliminated in the urine. It may be estimated that 1 g of ascorbic acid taken in four parts during the day (250 mg at breakfast, lunch, dinner, and in the evening) is as effective as 2 g taken at one time. Convenience may, however, justify the ingestion of the daily ascorbic acid at one time; for example, at breakfast. It is unlikely that there is any serious consequence of taking it in a single dose. The resistance to infection may well be determined by the lowest concentration in the blood and tissues, however, rather than the average concentration, so that regular ingestion is desirable.

A large quantity of ascorbic acid taken at one time has a laxative action, especially taken without food. It is probably desirable to take your ascorbic acid after a meal, rather than before the meal. If you seem to have problems with your digestion, it might be worth while to try taking your vitamin C as sodium ascorbate rather than ascorbic acid. It is almost tasteless, but when added to orange juice it gives it a slightly salty taste. A 50:50 mixture of ascorbic acid and sodium ascorbate is less acidic than ascorbic acid itself, and may be preferred by some people. It is available from some retail firms. Some people also find that timed-release vitamin C tablets are best for them.

Since human beings show biochemical individuality, there is the possibility that a person may respond in an unusual way to an increased intake of ascorbic acid. Because ascorbic acid is required as an essential nutrient, and all of our ancestors tolerated it for millions of years, it is very unlikely that anyone would have a serious allergic response to it. There is, however, a slight possibility of allergy to the filler, if tablets are taken. It is, of course, wise to increase or decrease the daily intake of this nutrient gradually.

A few months of experience should be enough to tell you whether the amount of ascorbic acid that you are ingesting approximates the desirable amount, the amount that provides protection against the common cold. If you are taking 1 g per day, and find that you have developed two or three colds during the winter season, it would be wise to try taking a larger daily quantity.

Also, if you are exposed to a cold, by having been in contact with a person suffering from a cold, or if you have become chilled by exposure or tired by overwork or lack of sleep, it would be wise to increase the amount of ascorbic acid ingested.

A convenient way of taking ascorbic acid is to stir the quantity desired, as fine crystals, in a glass of orange juice, where it quickly dissolves. One level teaspoonful is approximately 4 g (more accurately, 4.4 g), so that 1 g is obtained by taking one-quarter of a level teaspoonful of the crystals. The crystals may also be dissolved in tomato juice or cranberry juice, or simply in water, with sugar added if the acid taste is unpleasant. Tablets of ascorbic acid may, of course, be used.

The availability of ascorbic acid as fine crystals and as tablets is discussed in Appendix I.

HOW TO AMELIORATE A COLD

The regular use of ascorbic acid in the optimum daily amount appropriate to you as an individual human being may suffice to keep you from catching the common cold or influenza or other infection under most circumstances. But even if, under unusual circumstances, a cold begins to develop, there is still the possibility of ameliorating it or even stopping it by the use of ascorbic acid.

It is wise to carry some 1,000-mg tablets of ascorbic acid with you at all times. At the first sign that a cold is developing, the first feeling of scratchiness of the throat, or presence of mucus in the nose, or muscle pain or general malaise, begin the treatment by swallowing one or two 1,000-mg tablets. Continue the treatment for several hours by taking an additional tablet or two tablets every hour.

If the symptoms disappear quickly after the first or second dose of ascorbic acid, you may feel safe in returning to your usual regimen. If, however, the symptoms are present on the second day, the regimen should be continued, with the ingestion of 5 g to 20 g of ascorbic acid per day.

Régnier has pointed out (1968) that his observations indicate that when a cold is suppressed or averted by the use of an adequate amount of ascorbic acid the viral infection does not disappear at once, but remains suppressed, and that it is accordingly important that the vitamin-C regimen be continued for an adequate period of time. He recommends ingestion of about 4 g of ascorbic acid, in divided doses, per day for the first three or four days, dropping then to about 3 g for three or four days, then to 2 g per day, and then to 1 g per day.

It is not unreasonable that, because of individual variability, the suppression of the disagreeable manifestations of the common cold could be achieved for some people by a regimen involving the daily ingestion for a few days of a smaller amount of ascorbic acid, 1 g or 2 g per day, and that a larger amount, 10 g or 20 g per day, would be necessary for others.

It may be worth while to help control a cold by the topical application of a solution of sodium ascorbate, made by dissolving 3.1 g of sodium ascorbate in 100 ml of water. Braenden (1973), who has reported success in curing most colds or markedly alleviating the symptoms by this method, recommends introducing twenty drops of this solution into each nostril with an eye dropper. He has pointed out that in this way a local concentration of ascorbate a thousand times the value produced by oral administration can be reached.

Ascorbic acid is inexpensive and harmless, even when it is ingested in large amounts. A common cold, when it develops, may involve serious discomfort and suffering, inconvenience and reduced efficiency, and even disability for some days. Moreover, it may lead to the complications of more serious infections. It is accordingly better to overestimate the amount of ascorbic acid needed to control the cold than to underestimate it. A person with a chronic ailment should, of course, consult his physician about his ascorbic-acid intake.

The amount 1 g to 5 g per day of ascorbic acid is not large, compared with the amounts of other foods ingested daily. The recommended daily intake of protein by an adult is 50 g to 70 g or more, corresponding to between 1 g and 3 g of each of the eight essential amino acids. Carbohydrates and fats are required for energy. The average amount of carbohydrate ingested by an adult is about 300 g per day, and the average amount of fat is about 100 g per day.

It is recommended by responsible medical authorities that physicians not prescribe antibiotics, such as penicillin, for the common cold, Moreover, there is an additional hazard associated with the injection of an antibiotic, such as penicillin, that can be administered by mouth. Part of the additional hazard is that injections, if carried out with insufficient care, may introduce viruses that can cause diseases into the body. A somewhat larger dose of an antibiotic taken by mouth is often as effective as a dose given by injection.

You must not be disappointed if your physician at first expresses opposition to your use of ascorbic acid as recommended in this book. In the past the medical student has been taught little about vitamins and nutrition in medical school. Fortunately, physicians are now beginning to recognize the value of the vitamins and of orthomolecular therapy in general.

Ascorbic acid can be purchased retail, as fine crystals in 1-kilogram bottles, for about $10 per kilogram, at the present time 1976). Five hundred grams per year is the amount needed for the regimen described above as one that will avert or greatly ameliorate essentially all colds for many people. At $10 per kilogram, the cost of this regimen comes to $5 per year, as compared with $75 per year estimated in Chapter 1 as the value that might be placed on being essentially free of colds during the year.

If the use of ascorbic acid, as recommended above, were to become general, the price of ascorbic acid would decrease, so that the cost of a year's supply would probably drop as low as one dollar per person. The sum required to protect nearly all the American people against the common cold, two hundred million dollars per year, would then be far less than the amounts now being spent for aspirin and other drugs that are used in the effort to decrease somewhat the severity of the infections, and less than 2 percent of the estimate of 15 billion dollars made in Chapter 1 as representing the monetary damage done by colds in the United States.

VACCINATION AGAINST INFLUENZA

It is pointed out in Chapter 2 that some protection against influenza is provided by vaccination. The vaccine is usually prepared with killed virus that has been grown in fertilized eggs. Vaccination is said to be about 70 to 80 percent effective, and sometimes is accompanied by side effects. Because of possible side effects, it is usually recommended only for persons at high risk of infection.

In February 1976 there was an outbreak of influenza in a large military establishment in Fort Dix, New Jersey. One young serviceman, exhausted by his participation in strenuous exercises, died of pneumonia. Typing of the virus showed that about 500 of the 12,000 persons in the camp had been infected by a swine-influenza virus, given the name A/NJ/76, whereas some others had been infected by another virus, A/Victoria/75, which was then sweeping over the United States and

Europe. Although the virus A/NJ/76 seemed to have died out after infecting only 4 percent of the people in the camp, the resemblance of the virus to that of the 1918–1919 pandemic (Chapter 2) and the death by pneumonia of one person after a strenuous night-time military exercise while he was suffering from swine flu caused fears that another swine-flu epidemic might occur in 1976–1977. President Ford announced in March that $135 million had been appropriated by the Federal Government to support the preparation of vaccine by pharmaceutical companies in an amount great enough to permit essentially all of the people in the United States to be vaccinated.

Two of the companies, Merrell-National Laboratories and Merck Sharp and Dohme, are making killed whole-virus vaccine and two, Wyeth Laboratories and Parke-Davis and Company, are making split-virus vaccine, in which the killed virus particles are split in half. The two kinds are about equally effective. Some vaccines, called monovalent, are made with A/NJ/76 virus alone, and some, called bivalent, with both A/NJ/76 and A/Victoria/75 viruses.

Tests with influenza vaccines have shown a moderately high incidence of mild reactions. In one study with 6,000 healthy adults inoculated with influenza-A vaccine, influenza-B vaccine, or a mixture (Smith, Fletcher, and Wherry, 1975) about one third showed no symptoms, 50 percent complained of local pain, and 40 percent showed some general symptoms, with an incidence of days of absence from work attributed to the immunization only 1.1 per 100 persons. In approximately 16,500 injections only 2 patients had an acute reaction resembling an allergy. The results of studies of the response of about 1,000 children to the 1976 swine-flu vaccine were reported at a meeting at the National Institutes of Health on 21 June 1976. Many of the children six to ten years old showed reactions—transient fever, headache, muscle soreness—even with doses so small that two inoculations, two weeks apart, might be needed to confer immunity. The testing of children three to six years old will not be completed until October. There is the possibility that the program will be changed so as not to involve people under twenty-three years old except those of high risk because of respiratory disease or heart disease.

The possibility of serious side effects and resultant law suits asking for compensation has caused the insurance companies to refuse to provide insurance for manufacturers of the vaccines. These companies asked the Federal Government to provide this insurance and the Government has agreed to provide it. These actions have caused questions to be asked about the safety of the announced program, and it seems likely that it will be modified somewhat.

The question of how serious the threat of a pandemic really is has also been raised. During the last forty years the epidemics of influenza have shown remarkably little variation in their virulence. The high mortality in the 1918–1919 epidemic, especially among the younger adults, might have resulted from the malnutrition and other stresses at the end of a long war, causing the virus to be more than usually virulent and favoring the occurrence of secondary bacterial pneumonia (Francis, 1953; Stuart-Harris, 1976).

A study has been made of the virulence for man of the swine-flu virus A/NJ/76 in comparison with ten other strains of wild human influenza-A virus (Beare and Craig, 1976). The average clinical score for the persons inoculated with one or another of the ten human strains varied from 13.9 to 74.0, with average 41.3, and the score for the six persons inoculated with A/NJ/76 varied from 0 to 23, average 13.7. One of the six had no illness, one very mild, three mild, and one a moderate attack of influenza. The conclusion of the investigators was that the Fort Dix virus in its present form is less virulent in man than the established human influenza-A viruses but is a good deal more infectious and virulent than two Middle-West swine viruses, A/swine/Wisconsin/1/66 and A/swine/Manitoba/674/67, which they had tested previously.

From time to time restricted outbreaks of influenza caused by a virus that normally infects another species of animal occur. An example is the outbreak of an epidemic of human influenza in pigs in Taiwan in 1970 (Kundin, 1970), and another possible example is the observed illness of horses during the 1732 influenza epidemic in humans. The facts that the infection in Fort Dix affected only 4 percent of the persons in the camp and that no other cases of swine flu have been reported since the Fort Dix outbreak lend support to the suggestion by Stuart-Harris that the Fort Dix episode may be an isolated occurrence. It now seems quite unlikely that there will be a swine-flu epidemic, and there is now little justification for recommending mass vaccination.

THE CONTROL OF INFLUENZA

The measures to be taken for the prevention and treatment of influenza through use of vitamin C are essentially the same as for the common cold, as given in the first sections of this chapter. For most people the regular intake of 1 g or more per hour, should be begun. Also, a high intake of vitamin C should not be used as an excuse for continuing to work until exhaustion sets in. A person who may be contracting a cold should go to bed, rest for a few days, and take plenty of fluids along with his vitamin C, to have a much greater chance of avoiding serious illness.

If you have a fever for more than a couple of days, or a very high fever, be sure to call your physician.

A good intake of vitamin C should prevent a secondary bacterial infection from beginning. If it does begin, your physician can control it by a suitable regime with antibiotics. Some physicians, following Klenner, might inject large amounts of sodium ascorbate.

Persons with special risk, such as those with heart, lung, kidney, and certain metabolic diseases, including diabetes, may be advised to be vaccinated against influenza, as may also doctors, nurses, and others exposed to the virus to more than the usual extent. They should also take vitamin C; it will protect against the side effects of the vaccination, as well as against the disease.

If an attack of influenza begins and is not stopped by vitamin C, continue to take the vitamin in large amounts. It should make the attack a light one, of short duration.

CONCLUSION

Most people suffer from regular bouts with the common cold and occasional attacks of influenza. I believe that the application of a simple form of orthomolecular medicine, the use of ascorbic acid, can be effective in averting and ameliorating the common cold and influenza, and can contribute significantly to the control also of other diseases. I hope that this book will help in achieving this result.

Appendixes

How to Buy Vitamin C

Vitamin C is the substance L-ascorbic acid or one of its salts. Two of these salts, sodium ascorbate and calcium ascorbate, are present in some preparations; they are equally effective with ascorbic acid, when correction is made for the greater mass of the sodium atom or half of a calcium atom than of the hydrogen atom that is displaced. A 1,000-mg tablet of vitamin C may contain 1,000 mg of ascorbic acid or 1,125 mg of sodium ascorbate or 1,108 mg of calcium ascorbate—the vitamin-C activity is the same for all three.

Sometimes L-ascorbic acid is called natural ascorbic acid, the form that occurs in nature (in foodstuffs), to distinguish it from D-ascorbic acid, a closely related substance that does not have vitamin-C activity. You do not need to worry about whether you are buying vitamin C when you buy ascorbic acid, U.S.P. (United States Pharmacopeia); the inactive form is not on the market.

So-called synthetic ascorbic acid is natural ascorbic acid, identical with the vitamin C in oranges and other foods. The labels of some preparations of vitamin C emphasize that the tablets contain natural vitamin C or natural ascorbic acid in such a way as to suggest that this fact justifies a high price. You should not be taken in by this, because all vitamin-C preparations contain natural vitamin C.

The best way to buy vitamin C is to check the price and the content of vitamin C and then to get the most for your money. The best buy is pure crystalline L-ascorbic acid. It can be bought retail by mail from at least one pharmaceutical company, Bronson Pharmaceuticals, La Cañada, California, for less than $10 per kilogram (price in 1976). This amounts to 1¢ per day for an intake of 1 g per day. Pure sodium ascorbate and a 50:50 mixture of the acid and the sodium salt can also be purchased at a slightly higher price. A level teaspoonful is about $4\frac{1}{2}$ g. These pure substances have the advantage of not containing any filler, binder, or coloring or flavoring material, which might cause trouble for some people.

You must be careful not to be taken in by unscrupulous companies. After I had recommended pure vitamin-C crystals or powder in my book *Vitamin C and the Common Cold* I saw an advertisement for "Vitamin C Powder" at a price just under $10 per kilogram. I bought a bottle from the company, which was based in Kansas City, Missouri, and found in small print on the label the statement "Each level tablespoonful contains 500 mg ascorbic acid." A level tablespoonful is about 14 g. Accordingly the preparation contains only 36 g of ascorbic acid in a 1,000 g of powder; only one twenty-eighth of the powder is ascorbic acid, and the price is $280 per kilogram of vitamin C, not $10. I wrote to the FDA about this misrepresentation, and received in reply a statement that the FDA could do nothing about the matter. I then wrote to the Federal Trade Commission, which issued a cease-and-desist order on the company.

It is often convenient to have ascorbic acid available in

tablets. Tablets cost more than the pure substances because of the operation of making the tablets. The big tablets (1,000 mg) are a better buy than small tablets, and they have the advantage of not containing so much filler. They can be purchased for about $20 per thousand; that is, $20 per kilogram. Smaller tablets cost $25 or $30 per kilogram.

When you buy ascorbic acid, always calculate the price per kilogram. If it is much more than $10 for the pure substance or $20 to $25 for the tablets, don't buy, but go to another store.

If you belong to a cooperative market or shop at a large market, ask the manager to order some 1-kilogram bottles of Ascorbic Acid, fine crystals (or powder), and put them on the shelves for sale. He should be able to get it from the distributor at a wholesale price that permits the retail price to be about $10.00 for a 1 kilogram bottle. As mentioned above, tablets cost somewhat more.

Ascorbic acid in the form of fine crystals or crystalline powder kept in a brown or opaque white bottle is stable indefinitely, and can be kept for years. Dry tablets are also reasonably stable, and can be kept for years in a brown or opaque white bottle. Solutions of ascorbic acid may be oxidized when exposed to air and light. A solution of ascorbic acid in water may, however, be kept for several days in a refrigerator without significant oxidation. The solubility of ascorbic acid is high; water at ordinary temperatures can dissolve about one third its weight of ascorbic acid.

Everyone should ingest a varied diet, including green vegetables. Such a diet might provide 100 mg to 300 mg of ascorbic acid per day. Most meats contain very little ascorbic acid, less than 5 mg per 100 g (about 4 ounces). Organs such as brains, kidney, and liver, cooked, contain 10 mg to 30 mg per

100 g.* Orange juice contains about 50 mg per 100 g (one glass of fresh juice or freshly reconstituted frozen juice). Green vegetables (properly cooked), such as cabbage, spinach, broccoli, and mustard greens contain 30 mg to 90 mg per 100 g. Raw black currants and red or green peppers contain 200 mg to 350 mg per 100 g.

An ordinary good modern diet contains much less than the optimum amount of ascorbic acid. Thus for most people it is advisable to include additional ascorbic acid in the diet.

---

*It is probably by eating these organs that Eskimos get enough vitamin C to prevent scurvy when no plant foods are available.

Multivitamin Food Supplementation

In order to have the best of health, human beings must ingest an adequate quantity of each of the vitamins. The optimum intake no doubt varies from person to person. Probably almost everyone would benefit by supplementing his ordinary foods by the especially important foods called vitamins.

An easy way to carry out this supplementation is by taking a capsule or tablet containing a number of vitamins, a so-called multivitamin preparation. There is only one official multivitamin preparation listed in the United States Pharmacopeia. This preparation is called Decavitamin Capsules or Decavitamin Tablets, U.S.P. Each Decavitamin capsule or tablet (the two have the same composition of active substances) contains ten vitamins in the amounts shown in Table II-1.*

These amounts represent approximately the recommended dietary allowances of the ten vitamins, as given by the Food and Nutrition Board of the National Research Council. These

---

*These are the amounts given in earlier editions; the latest edition lists Decavitamin Capsules and Decavitamin Tablets but does not specify the amounts of vitamins in them.

TABLE II-1
Contents of Decavitamin Capsules or Tablets

Substance	Amount
Vitamin A	4,000 units
Vitamin D	400 units
Ascorbic Acid	75 mg
Thiamine (B_1)	1.0 mg
Riboflavin (B_2)	1.2 mg
Nicotinamide (Niacinamide)	10 mg
Folic Acid	0.25 mg
Pyridoxine (B_6)	2.0 mg
Calcium Pantothenate	5 mg
Cyanocobalamin (B_{12})	0.002 mg

recommended daily dietary allowances, given in the eighth report, 1974, and described as designed for the maintenance of good nutrition of practically all healthy people in the United States, are shown in Table II-2, for a 70-kilogram (154-pound) man.

Comparison of these amounts with the amounts in Decavitamin Capsules and Decavitamin Tablets shows that the U.S.P. preparations contain in two capsules or tablets the recommended daily allowance, or somewhat more, for all of the vitamins except vitamin E, which is not included in the Decavitamin Capsules or Tablets.

Multiple vitamins (multivitamins) in capsule or tablet form can be obtained in large drug stores and supermarkets. These food supplements are in packages with the composition given on the package. The composition is usually very nearly the same as the recommended daily dietary allowances, as listed

TABLE II-2
Daily dietary allowances recommended for a 154-pound man
by the Food and Nutrition Board of the National Research
Council

Substance	Amount
Vitamin A	5,000 International Units
Vitamin D	400 International Units
Ascorbic Acid	45 mg
Thiamine	1.5 mg
Riboflavin	1.6 mg
Nicotinic Acid (equivalent to the same amount of nicotinamide)	18 mg
Folic Acid	0.4 mg
Pyridoxine	2.0 mg
Cyanocobalamin	0.003 mg
Vitamin E	15 International Units

above, except that some of these preparations do not contain folic acid.

The cost of supplementing one's diet with two or three multivitamin capsules or tablets per day is not great. A bottle containing 1,000 capsules or 1,000 tablets can be purchased from some firms for about $6. (See Burack, *The New Handbook of Prescription Drugs,* 1970.) The cost in large drug stores and supermarkets is about the same; I have bought bottles containing 250 multivitamin tablets for $1.79. Supplementing one's diet by use of these multivitamin preparations accordingly costs only a few dollars per year.

The cost is much greater, five or ten times as much, if the vitamins are obtained with trade names or on prescription.

There is no advantage to the preparations with trade names, and no advantage to obtaining the vitamins by prescription.

Moreover, the cost of vitamins is in general considerably higher if they are obtained from special health-product sources. From a representative catalog of such a health-product firm I find that tablets essentially equivalent to Decavitamin Tablets U.S.P. are listed at $15 for 250, which is eight times the price mentioned above. As with vitamin C, it is wise to check the price and composition of any vitamin preparation carefully before buying it, in order that you not be misled into paying an exorbitant amount for it.

There is sound reason for believing that the recommended dietary allowances of most vitamins are significantly smaller than the optimum intakes. The values of thiamine, riboflavin, and niacin in a day's ration of raw natural plant foods (Table 3, in Chapter 8) are about three times the recommended dietary allowances of these three B vitamins. It seems reasonable from evolutionary considerations that the larger intakes of these vitamins may be closer to the optimum intakes, and there is in fact evidence that many people improve in health when they receive a dietary supplement containing larger amounts. One pharmaceutical company sells a Super-B tablet with the composition shown in Table II-3. These tablets are to be taken at the rate one per day or as directed by the physician.

Professor Roger J. Williams of the University of Texas has suggested a vitamin-mineral supplement for nutritional insurance, with the composition shown in Table II-4, as given in his book *Physicians Handbook of Nutritional Science* (1975). Tablets containing about one third of these amounts, except the vitamin K and cobalt, are manufactured by one company (Bronson), with the suggested dosage three tablets daily for

TABLE II-3
Contents of a Super-B Tablet

Substance	Amount
B_1 (thiamine mononitrate)	50 mg
B_2 (riboflavin)	50 mg
B_6 (pyridoxine hydrochloride)	50 mg
B_{12} (cyanocobalamin)	0.1 mg
Folic acid	0.4 mg
Biotin	0.4 mg
D-Calcium pantothenate	100 mg
Niacinamide	300 mg

adults and teenagers, two for children six to twelve years old, and one for younger children, or as directed by the physician.

Many persons are known to have serious genetic diseases involving physiological processes in the body in which vitamins take part. Control of the disease can sometimes be achieved by the intake of a very large amount of the appropriate vitamin. An example is the disease methylmalonicaciduria, discussed in Chapter 9. It is likely that most people are of such genetic character with respect to one or another of the vitamins as to require a somewhat larger amount of that vitamin for optimum health than other people do. It is difficult to detect such a need except by trial. It is especially important that people in poor health or borderline health be well nourished and that an effort be made to see whether or not they are benefitted by a high intake of vitamins (megavitamin treatment). Fortunately the water-soluble vitamins (vitamin C and the B vitamins) and also vitamin E have very low toxicity

TABLE II-4
Vitamin-mineral supplement suggested by Professor Williams

Amount	Substance	Amount	Substance
Vitamin A	7,500 units	Para-amino benzoic acid	30 mg
Vitamin D	400 units	Rutin	200 mg
Vitamin E	40 units	Calcuim	250 mg
Vitamin D (menadione)	2 mg	Phosphate	750 mg
Vitamin C	250 mg	Magnesium	200 mg
Thiamine	2 mg	Iron	15 mg
Riboflavin	2 mg		
Vitamin B_6	3 mg	Zinc	15 mg
Vitamin B_{12}	0.009 mg	Copper	2 mg
Niacinamide	20 mg	Iodine	0.15 mg
Pantothenic acid	15 mg	Manganese	5 mg
Biotin	0.3 mg	Molybdenum	0.1 mg
*Folic acid	0.4 mg	Chromium	1 mg
Choline	250 mg	Selenium	0.02 mg
Inositol	250 mg	Cobalt	0.1 mg

*More than the specified amount (about 2 mg) would be recommended if it were not for conflicting FDA regulations.

and few serious side effects. Care must be taken to avoid too great intake of vitamin A, vitamin D, and vitamin K.

Megavitamin treatment has been especially successful with schizophrenic patients, the principal vitamins used being niacin or niacinamide and vitamin C (Hoffer and Osmond, 1966; Hawkins and Pauling, 1973).

The literature about vitamins other than vitamin C in relation to disease is so extensive that it cannot even be abstracted in this book. Among the books in this field are those by Williams (1975), Cheraskin and Ringsdorf (1971, 1974), Rosenberg and Feldzamen (1974), and Passwater (1975).

It is wise not to rely entirely on such a dietary supplement for the essential foods. The essential amino acids are not required as a dietary supplement if an adequate supply of protein is ingested. Moreover, although it is believed that the most important essential nutrients for man are known, there is still the possibility that some have remained undiscovered. For this reason I agree with the specialists in nutrition that everyone should ingest a well-balanced diet, with a good amount of green vegetables, well prepared, and fresh fruits, such as oranges or grapefruit.

If we lived entirely on raw, fresh plant foods, as our ancestors did some millions of years ago, there would be no need for concern about getting adequate amounts of the essential foods, such as the vitamins. The vitamin content of foods is decreased by modern methods of processing and also by cooking. Accordingly it is often necessary to supplement the diet by ingesting additional amounts of these important foods, especially of ascorbic acid, for the reasons discussed earlier in this book.

There is some question whether the so-called bioflavonoids (vitamin P), which are substances extracted from the citrus fruits and other fruits, have any value in supplementing the protective power of ascorbic acid against the common cold. The bioflavonoids are effective in preventing fragility and permeability of the capillaries in guinea pigs, and have been used to some extent to decrease capillary fragility and permeability in humans. Vitamin P has not been included in an authoritative treatise, *Vitamins and Coenzymes*, by Wagner and

Folkers (1964). In the study by Franz, Sands, and Heyl (1956), in which it was found that subjects receiving ascorbic acid showed a more rapid improvement in their colds than those not receiving it, no difference was found between those receiving bioflavonoids, either with or without ascorbic acid, and those who did not receive bioflavonoids. Also, as mentioned in Chapter 6, Régnier (1968) reported that he began his studies by using both ascorbic acid and bioflavonoids, but soon observed that ascorbic acid alone seemed to be just as effective as the same amount of ascorbic acid with bioflavonoids.

I conclude that it is likely that bioflavonoids do not have much value in assisting in the control of the common cold, and accordingly need not be included in the regimen.

Good general nutrition, in addition to an adequate intake of ascorbic acid, is needed for protection against colds and other infections. It has been reported that the susceptibility to colds is decreased by an increase in the daily allowance of vitamin A for some people and of vitamin E for others. It is, however, ascorbic acid for which the ratio between the optimum intake and the usually recommended intake is the greatest and which is shown by the evidence to be the most important food for preventing colds.

Other Studies
of Ascorbic Acid
and the Common Cold

Many physicians have reported their observations that vitamin C seemed to have value in helping to control the common cold, as well as other diseases. The early reports of Korbsch (1938) and Ertel (1941) are mentioned in Chapter 6. Scheunert (1949) from a study of 2,600 factory workers in Leipzig reported that an intake of either 100 mg or 300 mg of vitamin C per day decreased the incidence of respiratory diseases and other diseases by about 75 percent. Bartley, Krebs, and O'Brien (1953) found that the mean length of colds in subjects deprived of ascorbic acid was twice as great as for subjects not deprived. Fletcher and Fletcher (1951) stated that supplements of 50 mg to 100 mg of ascorbic acid per day increased the resistance of children to infection. Some value of small amounts of ascorbic acid was reported also by Barnes (1961), Macon (1956), and Banks (1965, 1968). Marckwell (1947) stated that there was a 50-percent chance of stopping a cold if enough ascorbic acid were taken: 0.75 g at once, followed by 0.5 g every three or four hours, continuing on later days if needed. Bessel-Lorck (1959) found in a study of forty-six students in a ski camp in the mountains that those who received 1 g of vitamin C per day had only about half as much illness as those who received no vitamin C.

The controlled trials began in 1942, with the work of Glazebrook and Thomson and that of Cowan, Diehl, and Baker, discussed in Chapter 6. A number of other controlled trials have been carried out. Those of Ritzel (1961), Anderson, Reid, and Beaton (1972), Coulehan et al. (1974), and Sabiston and Radomski (1974) have been mentioned in Chapter 6 and several others are described below.

Anderson, Suranyi, and Beaton

A second double-blind study, with over 2,000 subjects, was carried out in Toronto (Anderson, Suranyi, and Beaton, 1974). In this very large study there were two placebo groups, one with 285 and the other with 293 subjects, and six ascorbic-acid groups (receiving various amounts), with 275 to 331 subjects. The study continued for three months.

A complication in the analysis of this study is presented by the fact that the results observed for the two placebo groups do not agree with one another. One placebo group had the greatest amount of illness of all eight groups, and the other had the smallest amount. The authors conclude that their observations are compatible with an effect of small magnitude (less than 20 percent) from both the prophylactic regimen (250 mg, 1 g, or 2 g of ascorbic acid per day) and the therapeutic regimen (4 g or 8 g on the first day of illness), with an effect of somewhat greater magnitude from the combined regimen (1 g per day and 4 g on the first day of illness). They state also that there was no evidence of side effects from the 1 g or 2 g of ascorbic acid per day and no evidence of a rebound increase in illness during the month following withdrawal of the daily vitamin supplement.

The authors give the amounts of illness per subject (days of symptoms, days indoors, days off work) relative to the first placebo group and also relative to the first plus the second. I have averaged these two sets of values, and have obtained 9 percent as the average decrease in amount of illness of the ascorbic-acid subjects. This value is uncertain, however. The great difference between the two placebo groups makes it likely that an error of some sort was made in this study.

Anderson, Beaton, Corey, and Spero

One of the best of the controlled studies is the third Toronto study (Anderson et al., 1975). Of the 488 subjects who completed the fifteen-week test 150 received a weekly 500-mg vitamin C tablet (two-thirds sodium ascorbate and one-third calcium ascorbate), 152 received a weekly 500-mg timed release capsule of ascorbic acid, and 145 received a placebo tablet with the same appearance and taste as the ascorbate tablet. In addition the subjects were instructed to take an extra tablet or capsule at the onset of any symptom of illness and, if symptoms persisted, to repeat the dose twice at four-hour intervals on the first day and once every twelve hours for up to four more days.

The investigators report for each of the three groups the average number of days of illness per subject with nine signs or symptoms—confined indoors, off work, nose running or plugged, throat soreness, chest soreness or tightness, felt feverish, cold and shivery, limbs aching and heavy, and mentally depressed, no ambition. This average was less for each of the two vitamin groups than for the placebo group for every one of the nine signs or symptoms, with ratios ranging from 62 to 98 percent. The averages of the nine values for the two vitamin groups, 75 and 78 percent, respectively, are nearly the same, and the investigators made other comparisons between the combined vitamin group (302 subjects) and the placebo group. The subjects in each of these two groups were divided into a high and a low subgroup in nine ways, according to age, sex, usual days indoors, contact with young children, frequency in crowds, daily juice, vitamin supplement, smoking, and episodes involving nasal symptoms. The average number of days indoors per subject for each of the eighteen vitamin subgroups was less than that for the corresponding placebo subgroup, with the ratio ranging from 48 percent (for episodes not involving nasal symptoms) to 87 percent.

The average number of days indoors per subject was 1.202 for the whole vitamin group and 1.610 for the placebo group, with a ratio of 75 percent, corresponding to 25 percent less illness for the vitamin group than for the placebo group. The investigators state that "subjects in both vitamin groups experienced less severe illness than subjects in the placebo group, with approximately 25 percent fewer days spent indoors because of illness." They point out that the results are similar to those obtained in their first study, in which they found 30 percent fewer days confined to home, with a larger intake of vitamin C (Anderson, Reid, and Beaton, 1972). They also mention that in each study as much protection against nonrespiratory illness as against respiratory illness was observed, and suggest again that large doses of ascorbic acid produce "a generalized nonspecific improvement in the host's ability to cope with infection (or possibly any type of stress?)." They express the opinion that "Taken in conjunction with the positive results reported by other investigators, there is now little doubt that the intake of additional vitamin C can lead to a reduced burden of 'winter illness'."

Charleston and Clegg

Charleston and Clegg (1972) carried out a fifteen-week study with ninety subjects in Glasgow. The forty-seven ascorbic-acid subjects (1 g per day) had an average of 0.94 colds, with average duration 3.5 days, corresponding to 3.29 days of illness per person, and the forty-three placebo subjects had an average of 1.86 colds, with an average duration of 4.2 days, corresponding to 7.81 days of illness per person. The observed decrease in amount of illness per person is accordingly 58 percent. The study was not double-blind, in that one investigator knew the identity of the subjects in the two groups.

Masek, Neradilova, and Hejda

Masek, Neradilova, and Hejda (1972) have reported the results of a double-blind study carried out over a period of four weeks with 2,535 coal miners in Czechoslovakia, 1,230 of whom (the workers in one mine) received a 100-mg tablet of ascorbic acid each day and 1,305 (the workers in another mine, nearby) a placebo. The amount of illness per person was 16 percent less for the ascorbic-acid subjects than for the placebo subjects. The average ascorbate concentration in the blood before the test was 4.5 mg per liter for each of the two groups; at the end of the test (four weeks) it was 4.0 mg per liter for the placebo group and 8.1 mg per liter for the vitamin group. A second test was carried out over a period of eight weeks with 1,100 workers in another mine, with alternate workers receiving 100 mg of the vitamins per day, the others nothing. The physician in charge of the men did not know which ones were receiving the vitamin. The decrease in amount of illness per person was 15 percent, essentially the same as the first test.

Elliott

A ten-week double-blind study of seventy crew members on a Polaris submarine was carried out by Elliott (1973). The thirty-seven subjects in the ascorbic-acid group received 2 g of ascorbic acid per day and the thirty-three control subjects received a placebo. There was no consistent difference between the two groups in the incidence of runny nose and sneezing. The average number of days of morbidity for hoarseness, sore throats, and coughs was 66 percent less for the vitamin-C subjects than for the placebo subjects.

Wilson, Loh, and Foster

Some double-blind studies involving students in boarding schools in Dublin have been reported by Wilson and his collaborators (1973). Their analysis is complicated by the

subdivision of colds into three somewhat over-lapping catego-
ries, catarrhal, toxic, and whole, and it has not been possible
for me to obtain from their reports a reliable value of the
difference in amount of illness of the vitamin-C groups and the
controls. The investigators reported that girls were significantly benefitted by an increased intake of ascorbic acid (200
mg or 500 mg per day) but that boys were not. It is interesting
and perhaps pertinent here that Coulehan et al. (1974) found a
signficant protective effect of vitamin C for the younger boys
and girls and for the older girls, but not for the older boys. For
the younger children and the older girls analysis of blood
samples showed no change in the ascorbate concentration for
the placebo groups and a pronounced rise for the vitamin-C
groups, but for the older boys there was the same rise (smaller
than for the younger children and older girls in the vitamin-C
groups) for both the vitamin-C group and the placebo group.
These observations indicate that the older boys exchanged
their tablets with one another. Swiss boys are probably as
mischievous as the Irish boys, but Ritzel outwitted them by
having them swallow their tablets under observation by the
physician.

Karlowski et al.

The results of a double-blind nine-months study with 190
employees of the National Institutes of Health have been
reported by Karlowski, Chalmers, Frenkel, Kapikian, Lewis,
and Lynch (1975). The study was well-designed and well-
executed except for the use of a poor placebo, easily distinguished from ascorbic acid by taste. Ascorbic acid, 1 g per day,

was taken by 101 subjects, of whom 57 also received an additional 3 g per day for the first five days of any illness, beginning, however, only after the subjects had returned to the pharmacy to have their symptoms and clinical observations recorded and to receive their supplemental capsules. A group of 46 received only placebo capsules, and a group of 43 received daily placebo capsules and ascorbic-acid supplementary capsules.

The reported average number of days of illness per person was 7.88 for the subjects who received 1 g of vitamin C per day and 10.01 for the 46 placebo subjects. The vitamin-C subjects thus had 21 percent less illness than the control group. A somewhat smaller decrease in illness was found for the group taking only supplemental ascorbic acid, 16 percent.

Although a placebo indistinguishable from the vitamin-C capsule was available to them, the investigators used one containing only milk sugar (lactose) and calcium stearate, easily identified as lacking the acid taste of ascorbic acid. Many of the subjects had tasted the contents of their capsules and correctly interpreted the taste. Much of the decreased illness was found in the subjects who learned in this way that they were receiving ascorbic acid. The investigators indicate in their paper that much of the apparent protective effect of ascorbic acid might be the result of a psychological effect, the power of suggestion. I doubt that such psychological effects can operate significantly in a large population over periods of several months. In any case, the National Institutes of Health study cannot be described as one of the best.

Karlowski et al. conclude "that ascorbic acid had at best only a minor influence on the duration and severity of colds, and that the effects demonstrated might be explained well by a break in the double blind." They also say that "the effects of ascorbic acid on the number of colds seem to be nil," and this statement was quoted in the AMA press release of 10 March 1975, referred to in Chapter 12, without the additional information about the number of colds given by Karlowski et al. In fact, the group receiving prophylactic ascorbic acid had 16 percent fewer colds than the control group.

Dahlberg, Engel, and Rydin

A double-blind study was carried out by Dahlberg, Engel, and Rydin with 2,525 Swedish soldiers in a camp in northern Sweden during ninety days in 1941. The ascorbic-acid subjects (1,266) received an average of 90 mg per day, and the control subjects (1,259) received a placebo. Examination of the tables in their paper shows that the incidence of colds in the ascorbic-acid subject was 8 percent less than in the control subjects, and the incidence of infectious diseases of all sorts was 10.0 percent less. The numbers of days of illness per person were recorded but are not given in the paper. The diseases were 5 percent less severe in the ascorbic-acid group than in the placebo group. The differences are not statistically significant, and the investigators themselves concluded that the ascorbic acid had shown no protective effect. Their tables show, however, that the small added intake of ascorbic acid (average 90 mg per day) is associated with an apparent decrease in amount of illness of about 14 percent.

Franz, Sands, and Heyl

A double-blind three-months study with 195 mg of vitamin C per day was reported in 1956 by Franz, Sands, and Heyl. The subjects were eighty-nine volunteer medical students and nurses at Dartmouth Medical School. They were divided, in a random way, into four groups, three of twenty-two subjects and one of twenty-three subjects. One group received tablets containing ascorbic acid, the second ascorbic acid and a bioflavonoid (naringin), the third a placebo, and the fourth naringin only. The daily amount of ascorbic acid was 205 mg and that of the bioflavonoid was 1,000 mg. Symptoms of colds were systematically recorded. The results for the bioflavonoid groups, with or without ascorbic acid, were the same as for the corresponding groups without bioflavonoid. The authors con- cluded that the administration of a bioflavonoid had effect neither on the incidence or the cure of colds nor on the ascorbic-acid level of the blood. There were fourteen colds in the groups receiving vitamin C or vitamin C plus bioflavonoid (forty-four subjects), and fifteen colds in the groups receiving placebo or placebo plus bioflavonoid (forty-five subjects). The colds in the vitamin-C subjects were of short duration, only one lasting longer than five days, whereas for the placebo subjects eight of the fifteen colds lasted longer than five days. From the detailed observations of day-by-day symptoms in another investigation (Abbott et al., 1968) I estimated the average duration of the 5-days-or-less colds to be 3.6 days and of the others to be 7.8 days. The observations of Franz, Sands, and Heyl then correspond to 36 percent less illness per person for the vitamin-C subjects than for the placebo subjects.

A second study was carried out in Glasgow by Clegg and Macdonald (1975). The study was double-blind and lasted fifteen weeks, with 77 subjects (126 men and 75 women) taking 1 g of ascorbic acid per day and 80 taking a placebo. The amount of illness was 8 percent less for the ascorbic-acid subjects than for the controls. It is interesting, in connection with the statement made by Wilson et al, about boys and girls in Dublin, that in this Glasgow study the men showed no protection (actually 1 percent greater amount of illness), whereas there was 22 percent protection for the women.*

RESULTS OF THE CONTROLLED STUDIES

The values of the decreases in the amount of illness per person in the ascorbic-acid subjects relative to the control subjects for fourteen controlled trials, described in Chapter 6 and the preceding sections of this appendix, are given in Table III-1. These fourteen trials comprise all of the trials known to me that meet certain specifications. One is that ascorbic acid be given regularly over a period of time to subjects who were not ill at the start of the trial, with the subjects selected from a larger population by some randomizing method. The study by Masek et al. (1972) is not included because the vitamin-C subjects were the workers in one mine and the placebo subjects were those in another, where the conditions affecting the health of the workers might have been either better or worse. In all but one of the studies a placebo, a tablet or capsule closely resembling the vitamin-C tablet or capsule, was given to the control subjects. The one exception was the carefully conducted and thorough study by Glazebrook and Thomson (1942) in which ascorbic acid was added to the food (cocoa or

---

*Clegg and Macdonald also reported a 40-percent protective effect by 1 g of D-isoascorbic acid, an isomer of L-ascorbic acid that does not protect against scurvy but it similar to it in some properties. The significance of this observation is not yet clear.

TABLE III-1
Summary of results of controlled studies of amount
of illness per subject in ascorbic-acid subjects
relative to placebo subjects

Study	Amount of decrease in illness per person
*Glazebrook, Thomson (1942)	50%
*Cowan, Diehl, Baker (1942)	31%
*Dahlberg, Engel, Rydin (1944)	14%
*Franz, Sands, Heyl (1956)	36%
Ritzel (1961)	63%
Anderson, Reid, Beaton (1972)	32%
Charleston, Clegg (1972)	58%
Elliott (1973)	44%
Anderson, Suranyi, Beaton (1974)	9%
Coulehan et al. (1974)	30%
Sabiston, Radomski (1974)	68%
Karlowski et al. (1975)	21%
*Anderson et al. (1975)	25%
Clegg, Macdonald (1975)	8%
Average	35%

*70 to 200 mg per day, average 31%; others, average 40%

milk) of one or more of the seven divisions of boys that were
served in seven different places in the dining hall. The study by
Wilson et al. (1973) is not listed in Table III-1 because of the
difficulty of determining from their papers the decrease in the
amount of illness.

The average of the fourteen values of the decrease in the
amount of illness per person is 35 percent. For the five studies
in which only 70 mg to 200 mg of ascorbic acid per day was

given the average is 31 percent, and for the nine in which 1 g per day or more was given it is 40 percent. We may conclude that even a small added intake of vitamin C, 100 mg or 200 mg per day, has considerable value, and that a larger intake probably has somewhat more value.

CONTROLLED STUDIES OF THE EFFECT OF VITAMIN C TAKEN AFTER A COLD HAS STARTED

In Chapter 6 it is mentioned that Régnier (1968) carried out a controlled trial that led him to the conclusion that a few grams of ascorbic acid taken as soon as possible after a cold has begun would avert 90 percent of the colds. A few other studies of this kind have been carried out. Tebrock, Arminio, and Johnston reported in 1956 that they had tested the value of ascorbic acid, with or without bioflavonoids, in shortening the period of illness with the common cold. The amount of ascorbic acid administered was very small—only 200 mg per day for three days, beginning when the patient reported that he had a cold. Nearly 2,000 patients were studied, with half of them receiving ascorbic acid (total amount 0.6 g) and the other half receiving a placebo or a bioflavonoid capsule. No difference in the duration of the colds was observed. The amount of ascorbic acid used was very much smaller than the amount used by Régnier. Even nearly 3 g per day may not be effective if the treatment is delayed until after the cold has begun. Cowan and Diehl (1950) reported no therapeutic effect when the ingestion of ascorbic acid was delayed until the cold was begun and was continued for only three days (2.66 g the first and second days. 1.33 g the third day). A similar lack of effectiveness of 3 g per day, starting after the cold had developed, was also reported by a group of seventy-eight British physicians (Abbott et al, 1968). It is likely that for most people an intake of 1 g or 2 g per hour, beginning at the first symptom of illness, will stop most attacks of the common cold or influenza, but controlled trials of these larger amounts other than that of Régnier have not yet been reported.

STUDIES WITH VIRUS-INDUCED COLDS

Many authorities quote, as the basis of their statements that vitamin C has no value in protecting against the common cold and influenza, the 1967 paper by Walker, Bynoe, and Tyrrell, of the Common Cold Research Unit in Salisbury, England, where the common cold has been studied since 1946. These investigators reported observations on tissue cultures, mice, and human volunteers, and concluded that "there is no evidence that the administration of ascorbic acid has any value in the prevention or treatment of colds produced by five known viruses." Of the ninety-one human volunteers, forty-seven received a placebo. They were all inoculated with cold viruses (rhinoviruses, influenza B virus, or B814 virus) on the third day. In each of the two groups (forty-seven in the ascorbic-acid group, forty-four in the control group), eighteen developed colds. There was no significant difference in the severity and duration of the colds.

The number of subjects, ninety-one in the two groups, was not great enough to permit a statistically significant test of a difference as large as 30 percent in the incidence of colds in the two groups to be made, although a difference of 40 percent, if it had been observed, would have been reported as statistically significant (probability of observation in a uniform population equal to 5 percent). The incidence of colds observed in the subjects receiving ascorbic acid (18/47) was 6 percent less than that in the control group (18/44) and the average number of days of illness was 9 percent less. Those differences are not statistically significant, and the observation does not rule out the possibility of a considerably larger protective effect. Also, this observation does not prove that somewhat larger amounts than 3 g per day would not be effective.

Moreover, the design of their study had a serious flaw (Pauling, 1976c). The administration of tablets was stopped an average of three days after the onset of the colds, and the colds lasted an average of five days longer. We know that when a large intake of ascorbic acid is suddenly stopped, the concentration of the vitamin in the blood drops for a few days to an abnormally low level, presumably because the high intake has induced the formation of increased amounts of enzymes that help convert the ascorbic acid into other substances (Chapter 11, the rebound effect). This abnormally low concentration of ascorbic acid decreases the effectiveness of the mechanisms of protection and may lead to exacerbation of the viral infection and the development of a secondary bacterial infection, as reported by Régnier. If Walker and his co-workers had not stopped the ascorbic-acid therapy after three days, the colds of their ascorbic-acid subjects might have had a much shorter duration. As mentioned above, Franz, Sands, and Heyl reported that for their ascorbic-acid group only 7 percent of the colds remained uncured or unimproved after five days, compared with 53 percent for their placebo group. For these several reasons, the study by Walker and associates cannot be accepted as providing significant evidence that ascorbic acid has no value in controlling the common cold and influenza. It would be well worth while for the investigators in the Common Cold Research Unit to carry out another controlled trial, with better design—a large amount of ascorbic acid, continued until the colds are over—but for nine years the Unit has refrained from making any more studies with vitamin C.

Ascorbic Acid
and Other Diseases

In addition to the common cold and influenza, many other diseases have been reported to be controlled to some extent by an increased intake of ascorbic acid. Viral and bacterial diseases that have been mentioned earlier in this book include viral pneumonia, hepatitis, poliomyelitis, tuberculosis, measles, mumps, chicken pox, viral orchitis, viral meningitis, shingles, fever blisters and cold sores, and canker sores. Topical application is sometimes of value, such as the use of nose drops of a solution of sodium ascorbate, mentioned in Chapter 14. Another example is treatment of cold sores on the lips or canker sores in the mouth by applying pure ascorbic acid as powder or fine crystals; the sores usually dry up in a few hours. Warts, which are also caused by a herpes virus, sometimes disappear when treated with a salve containing ascorbic acid.

It is, of course, astonishing that anyone would contend that a substance might be helpful to you no matter what disease you are suffering from. Nevertheless, the evidence is strong that vitamin C is such a substance. Vitamin C is not a wonder drug, a drug that cures a particular disease. It is instead a substance that participates in almost all of the chemical reactions that take place in our bodies, and is required for many of them. Our bodies can fight disease effectively only when we have in our organs and body fluids enough vitamin C to enable our natural protective mechanisms to operate effectively. This amount is much larger than the amount provided by our food, and it is much larger than the amount that has been recommended by the authorities in medicine and nutrition in the past. The evidence is so strong, however, that the authorities are now being forced to change their recommendations.

In one of their discussions of ascorbic acid in relation to cancer Cameron and Pauling (1974) list some of the ways in which an increased intake of this vitamin improves the effectiveness of the operation of the natural protective mechanisms of the body. One is the increase in strength of connective tissue and cell membranes because of the increased amount of the important structural protein collagen that is synthesized; ascorbic acid is required for the synthesis of collagen. Another is the increased effectiveness of leucocytes in attacking bacteria and malignant cells when the concentration of ascorbate is increased (Hume and Weyers, 1973). An important function of vitamin C has only recently been reported, by Yonemoto, Chretien, and Fehniger (1976). They found, with human subjects, that an intake of 5 g of ascorbic acid per day significantly increased the rate at which new lymphocyte cells are made, and an intake of 10 g per day had an even greater effect. Increased production of lymphocytes provides additional protection against infections and other threats to the body; in particular, Yonemoto et al. point out that it is known that cancer patients who make lymphocytes at a high rate have a greater chance for survival than those who make these cells at a low rate.

Vitamin C is also involved in the synthesis and release of the adrenocortical and pituitary hormones. Part of its effectiveness against stressful situations may be through a mechanism involving hormones.

The direct antiviral and antibacterial action of ascorbic acid may be of considerable importance in providing protection against many diseases. An example of a disease that has stubbornly resisted efforts to control it is leprosy. Recent studies have shown the presence in the patients of a defect in the functioning of their white cells, both lymphocytes and T-cells. Bacteriological studies and studies of mouse leprosy in mice suggested that vitamin C might be of value in controlling human leprosy, and promising results have been reported from the treatment of one patient with 1.5 g of ascorbic acid per day; an extensive trial, however, has not yet been carried out (Matsuo, et al, 1975; Skinsnes and Matsuo, 1976).

VITAMIN C AND SURGERY

The facts that ascorbic acid is required for the synthesis of collagen and that wounds in scorbutic persons fail to heal suggested that people undergoing surgery should receive an increased amount of vitamin C, and many surgeons order the administration of the vitamin to surgical patients. Several investigators have reported that surgical wounds do not heal in patients whose blood plasma concentration of ascorbate is less than 2 mg per liter, corresponding to an intake of less than 20 mg per day (references are given in the reviews by Schwartz,

1970). One patient with bilateral hernia and plasma concentration only 0.9 mg per liter was given 100 mg of ascorbic acid per day after the herniorrhaphy on one side, and after the second operation he was given 1,100 mg per day. The skin and fascia wounds on the first side healed poorly, whereas those on the second side healed well, with breaking strength three to six times that for the first side (Bartlett, Jones, and Ryan, 1942). It is likely that the amount 750 mg per day given by many surgeons to their patients is less than the optimum amount. A number of studies on the value of a high intake of ascorbic acid in promoting wound healing and preventing surgical shock are mentioned by Stone (1972), and a number of cases in which patients who received several grams of the vitamin per day and experienced unusually rapid wound healing and convalescence after surgery have been reported to me. Some surgeons now add 5 g of sodium ascorbate or more to each liter of intravenous fluid, in addition to giving extra vitamin C to the patient before the operation. Dr. Morishige, chief surgeon of Fukuoka Hospital, Fukuoka, Japan, now gives 10 g per day to each surgical patient.

Although no carefully controlled study has been reported of the effect on surgical patients of an intake of several grams of ascorbic acid per day, there is little doubt that it is beneficial, and it is likely that before long 10 g per day will be ordered for their patients by all surgeons. Although controlled studies have not yet been reported, observations by some physicians indicate that provision of ascorbic acid decreases the amount of postsurgical pain, decreases the time required for resumption of normal bodily functions, accelerates the healing of the surgical wounds, and decreases by several days the length of the period of hospitalization.

VITAMIN C AND HEART DISEASE

Cardiovascular disease, disease of the heart and blood vessels, constitutes the principal cause of death. During recent years it has become evident that nutritional and environmental factors are important in determining incidence of cardiovascular disease. Cigarette smoking is one of the most important ones. The average cigarette smoker, who smokes one pack a day, has at each age twice the chance of incurring heart disease and of dying of heart disease as the average nonsmoker.

Unsaturated fatty substances play an important part in the functioning of our biochemical machinery and in cell membranes and other tissues. These substances are converted by oxidation into peroxides that are harmful. Vitamin C and vitamin E are natural antioxidants. An increased intake of these vitamins provide protection against cardiovascular disease. Vitamin E may be the more important of these two natural antioxidants, but vitamin C is also important. A proper intake of vitamin C and vitamin E may help to prevent premature aging, especially if one's diet is rich in polyunsaturated fats.

Cholesterol is an important substance. Human beings manufacture about 1,000 mg per day, and it is destroyed at a somewhat greater rate, because in addition to the 1,000 mg manufactured in the cells of our body we obtain some cholesterol in foods. People with a high cholesterol concentration in the blood have been reported to have a higher incidence of cardiovascular disease than those with a lower concentration, and during the last twenty-five years there has been an effort to decrease the amount of cholesterol ingested with food.

An egg, for example, contains about 250 mg of cholesterol, which is present in the yolk. Animal fat, present in meat, also contains cholesterol. It is for this reason that the consumption of eggs and animal fat is decreased in a low-cholesterol diet.

It has been found that an increased intake of ascorbic acid decreases the concentration of cholesterol in the blood (Ginter, 1970, 1973, 1975; Spittle, 1971). Ginter gave twenty-four subjects, aged forty to seventy-five years, 1 g of ascorbic acid per day for six months. These subjects were selected as having a moderately high cholesterol level, averaging 253 mg per deciliter. After six months during which they received 1 g of ascorbic acid per day their average cholesterol level had dropped to 210 mg per deciliter. Control subjects who did not receive added ascorbic acid showed a slight increase, by 12 mg per deciliter. An increase of another vitamin, nicotinic acid, has also been shown to cause a decrease in the cholesterol level by about 50 mg per deciliter (Altschul et al., 1955).

The importance of an increased intake of ascorbic acid, in comparison with a decreased intake of cholesterol, can be made with use of the observation that adding one egg per day to the diet produces an average increase of 8 mg per deciliter in the concentration of cholesterol in the blood. From the observation of a decrease by 43 mg per deciliter on intake of 1 g of ascorbic acid per day, we may conclude that to take 1 g of vitamin C per day is as valuable in controlling the cholesterol concentration as to eliminate five eggs per day from the diet. It is hard to understand why the American Heart Association and the National Institutes of Health recommend strongly that the intake of eggs be decreased, but make no mention of the value of an increased intake of vitamin C.

There is another nutritional factor that is important with respect to heart disease. This factor is sugar—ordinary white sugar, raw sugar, brown sugar, unrefined sugar, or honey.

Until the last two hundred years the carbohydrate that human beings ingested was largely starch, together with a little honey. Starch is made of the simple sugar glucose, whereas ordinary sugar, sucrose, is a disaccarhide, consisting of a glucose residue and a fructose residue attached together. The average intake of sucrose in the United States is now 100 pounds per year, whereas one hundred and fifty years ago it was only about 2 pounds per year. The result is that the intake of fructose, which formerly came from honey and fruits, has increased from about 8 g per day to 80 g per day. Our bodies are not accustomed to handling this large amount of fructose, and it is not surprising that the high sugar intake causes trouble for us.

Winitz et al. (1964, 1970) carried out a careful study with eighteen subjects, who were inmates in a locked institution, without access to other food, during the whole period of the study, about six months. They were given a diet in which the carbohydrate consisted only of polymers of glucose. It was found that their serum cholesterol decreased rapidly from an average of 227 mg per deciliter to 160 mg per deciliter. When some of the glucose was replaced by an equivalent amount of sucrose it rose to its initial value. There is no doubt that the fructose half of the sucrose molecule is responsible for the higher level of serum cholesterol. Yudkin (1972) has made a study of the intake of sugar in relation to the incidence of coronary heart disease. From this study he concluded that persons who ingest 160 pounds of sugar or more per year have sixteen times the chance at each age of developing coronary heart disease than those who ingest 60 pounds per year or less.

From these observations the conclusion may be drawn that to decrease your chance of incurring cardiovascular disease you should decrease the intake of sugar, and also ingest a proper amount of vitamin C and vitamin E.

VITAMIN C AND CANCER

The apparently random way in which cancer strikes suggests that the natural defense mechanisms of the body play an important part in providing protection against it. If these defense mechanisms could be enhanced to maximum efficiency, a striking improvement in the control of the disease would result. The involvement of ascorbic acid in the natural defense mechanisms is now known to be so great that we may hope that a really significant control of cancer might be achieved by the proper use of ascorbic acid. Several epidemiological studies have shown a definite negative correlation between cancer and the intake of vitamin C. Persons with a higher intake, usually around 100 mg to 200 mg per day, have a much smaller age-corrected incidence of cancer than those with a smaller intake, equal to the recommended dietary allowance of 45 mg per day. Although carefully controlled studies of the effect of the optimum daily intake of 1 g to 10 g have not yet been made, I have estimated that the probability of incurring cancer at a given age might be decreased to one quarter of its present value if people were to take regularly the optimum amount, between 1 g and 10 g per day for most people.

Another way in which ascorbic acid can contribute to the control of cancer is by giving it to patients who have developed cancer. Irwin Stone in his 1972 book discusses the early papers by physicians who reported some success in the treatment of cancer by increasing the intake of ascorbic acid. Progress in this field in recent years is to be attributed largely to Ewan Cameron, a Scottish surgeon. In 1966 Cameron published a book, with the title *Hyaluronidase and Cancer,* in which he discussed the important part that the resistance of the host could play in controlling the growth of a malignant tumor. He pointed out that the malignant tumor infiltrates the surrounding tissues, and that one of the mechanisms that it uses to weaken the surrounding tissues is to synthesize an enzyme, hyaluronidase, that attacks the intercellular cement in the surrounding tissues. Over a period of several years he attempted to find a treatment with hormones that would control the action of this enzyme and slow down the growth of the tumor, but without success. Since an increased intake of ascorbic acid is known to strengthen the intercellular cement, in part by promoting the growth of collagen fibrils, he began in November 1971 a test of the value of supplemental ascorbate in the supportive treatment of cancer. The results obtained in fifty patients have been reported in his paper on a clinical trial of high-dose sodium ascorbate supplement in advanced human cancer (Cameron, Campbell, 1974; Cameron Campbell, and Jack, 1975). In a study of 100 patients with "untreatable" cancer who received 10 g of sodium ascorbate and 1,000 matched controls who were treated in the same way except for not receiving sodium ascorbate it was found that the average survival time of the ascorbate-treated patients was more than four times that for the controls, and in a significant percentage of them the disease seems to have been completely controlled (Cameron and Pauling, 1976). Additional studies are now being made.

The possible mechanisms of action of ascorbic acid against cancer have been discussed by Cameron and Pauling (1973, 1974). One important one is the stimulation of the natural immune mechanism. It is known that the probability of a favorable outcome for the cancer patient increases with an increase in the rate with which his body is able to manufacture lymphocytes. It has been shown recently by Yonemoto et al. (1976) that an intake of 5 g or 10 g of ascorbic acid per day increases greatly the rate of synthesis of the lymphocytes, which are then increasingly able to attack and destroy the malignant cells. The requirement of ascorbic acid for the synthesis of collagen, a principal component of fibrous tissue, suggests that with an increased intake of this vitamin the malignant tumor might be walled off. In 1974 Cameron and Pauling discussed this possibility in the following words: "On these grounds alone, an adequate supply of ascorbic acid would seem to be essential to sustain an effective stromal reaction, and to potentiate the latent ability of the host to encapsulate the malignant process in a relatively impermeable barrier of dense fibrous tissue. Thus the dietary availability of ascorbic acid might be the determining factor in converting a 'soft', cellular, rapidly proliferating, highly invasive neoplasm with minimal stromal response into a 'hard', contained, encapsulated, scirrhous tumor with restricted growth and limited invasiveness." There is now some reason to believe that by the use of the proper amount of ascorbic acid some malignant tumors can be changed in such a way as to cause them to disappear or to permit their complete removal by surgical intervention. The National Cancer Institute and other agencies have been reluctant to support investigations on the role of vitamin C and other vitamins in providing protection against and treatment of cancer, but it is likely that great progress will be made along these directions during the next few years.

References

Abbott, P.; seventy-seven others (1968) Ineffectiveness of Vitamin C in Treating Coryza. *The Practitioner* 200: 442–445.

Abraham, S.; Lowenstein, F. W.; Johnson, C. L. (1976) Dietary Intake and Biochemical Findings (preliminary), *First Health and Nutrition Examination Survey, United States,* 1971–1972. Department of Health, Education, and Welfare Publication No. (HRA) 76-1219-1.

Adams, J. M. (1967) *Viruses and Colds: The Modern Plague.* American Elsevier Publishing Company, New York.

Albanese, P. (1947) Treatment of Respiratory Infections With High Doses of Vitamin C. *El Dia Medico* 19: 1738–1740.

Altman, P. L. (1971) [Untitled.] *New York Times,* July 11.

Altman, P. L.; Dittmer, D. S. (1968) *Metabolism.* Federation of American Societies for Experimental Biology, Bethesda, Maryland.

Altschul, R.; Hoffer, A.; Stephan, J. D. (1955) Influence of Nicotinic Acid on Serum Cholesterol in Man. *Archives of Biochemistry* 54: 558–559.

Anderson, T. W.; Beaton, G. H.; Corey, P. N.; Spero, L. (1975) Winter Illness and Vitamin C: The Effect of Relatively Low Doses. *Canadian Medical Association Journal* 112: 823–826.

Anderson, T. W.; Reid, D. B. W.; Beaton, G. H. (1972) Vitamin C and the Common Cold: A Double Blind Trial. *Canadian Medical Association Journal* 107: 503–508.

Anderson, T. W.; Suranyi, G.; Beaton, G. H. (1974) The Effect on Winter Illness of Large Doses of Vitamin C. *Canadian Medical Association Journal* 111: 31–36.

Andrewes, C. (1965) *The Common Cold.* W. W. Norton & Company, New York.

Anonymous (1967) Ascorbic Acid and the Common Cold. *Nutrition Reviews* 25: 228–231.

Anonymous (1969) C, the Vitamin With Mystique. *Mademoiselle,* November, p. 189.

Anonymous (1971) Vitamin C, Linus Pauling, and the Common Cold. *Consumer Reports,* February, pp. 113–114.

Anonymous (1976) Is Vitamin C Really Good for Colds? *Consumer Reports,* February, pp. 68–70.

Baetgen, D. (1961) Ergebnisse der Behandlung der Hepatitis epidemica im Kindersalter mit hohen Dosen Ascorbinsäure in den Jahren 1957/58. *Medizinische Monatsschrift* 15: 30–36.

Banks, H. S. (1965) Common Cold: Controlled Trials. *The Lancet* 2: 790.

Banks, H. S. (1968) Controlled Trials in the Early Antibiotic Treatment of Colds. *The Medical Officer* 119: 7–10.

Barnes, F. E., Jr. (1961) Vitamin Supplements and the Incidence of Colds in High School Basketball Players. *North Carolina Medical Journal* 22: 22–26.

Bartlett, M. K.; Jones, C. M.; Ryan, A. E. (1942) Vitamin C and Wound Healing. II. Ascorbic Acid Content and Tensile Strength of Healing Wounds in Human Beings: *The New England Journal of Medicine* 226: 474–481.

Bartley, W.; Krebs, H. A.; O'Brien, J. R. P. (1953) *Medical Research Council Special Report Series* No. 280, Her Majesty's Stationery Office, London.

Beadle, G. W.; Tatum, E. L. (1941) Genetic Control of Biochemical Reactions in Neurospora. *Proceedings of the National Academy of Sciences U.S.A.* 27: 499–506.

Beare, A. S.; Craig, J. W. (1976) Virulence for Man of a Human

Influenza-A Virus Antigenically Similar to "Classical" Swine Viruses. *The Lancet* 2: 4–5.

Belfield, W. O.; Stone, I. (1975) Megascorbic Prophylaxis and Megascorbic Therapy: A New Orthomolecular Modality in Veterinary Medicine. *Journal of the International Academy of Preventive Medicine* 2: 10–26.

Bessel-Lorck, C. (1959) Erkältungs prophylaxe bei Jugendlichen im Skilager. *Medizinische Welt* 44: 2126–2127.

Bietti, G. B. (1967) Further Contributions on the Value of Osmotic Substances as Means to Reduce Intra-Ocular Pressure. *Ophthalmological Society of Australia* 26: 61–71.

Boissevain, C. H.; Spillane, J. H. (1937) Effect of Synthetic Ascorbic Acid on the Growth of Tuberculosis Bacillus. *American Review of Tuberculosis* 35: 661–662.

Bourne, G. H. (1946) The Effect of Vitamin C on the Healing of Wounds. *Proceedings of the Nutrition Society* 4: 204–211.

Bourne, G. H. (1949) Vitamin C and Immunity. *British Journal of Nutrition* 2: 346–356.

Braenden, O. J. (1973) The Common Cold: A New Approach. *International Research Communications System* 7: 12.

Brandt, R.; Guyer, K. E.; Banks, W. L., Jr. (1974) A Simple Method to Prevent Vitamin C Interference with Urinary Glucose Determinations. *Clinica Chimica Atca* 51: 103–104.

Brewer, T. H. (1966) *Metabolic Toxemia of Late Pregnancy: A Disease of Malnutrition.* Charles C. Thomas, Springfield, Illinois.

Briggs, M. H.; Garcia-Webb, P.; Davies, P. (1973) Urinary Oxalate and Vitamin-C Supplements. *The Lancet* 2: 201.

Burack, R. (1970) *The New Handbook of Prescription Drugs, Official Names, Prices, and Sources for Patient and Doctor.* Pantheon Books, New York.

Burns, J. J.; Mosbach, E. H.; Schulenberg, S. (1954) Ascorbic Acid Synthesis in Normal and Drug-treated Rats. *Journal of Biological Chemistry* 207: 679–687.

Cameron, E. (1966) *Hyaluronidase and Cancer.* Pergamon Press, Ltd., Oxford.

Cameron, E.; Campbell, A. (1974) The Orthomolecular Treatment of Cancer. II. Clinical Trial of High-Dose Ascorbic Acid Supplements in Advanced Human Cancer. *Chemico-Biological Interactions* 9: 285–315.

Cameron, E.; Campbell, A.; Jack, T. (1975) The Orthomolecular Treatment of Cancer. III. Reticulum Cell Sarcoma: Double Complete Regression Induced by High-dose Ascorbic Acid Therapy. *Chemico-Biological Interactions* 11: 387–393.

Cameron, E.; Pauling, L. (1973) Ascorbic Acid and the Glycosaminoglycans: An Orthomolecular Approach to Cancer and Other Diseases. *Oncology* 27: 181–192.

Cameron, E.; Pauling, L. (1974) The Orthomolecular Treatment of Cancer. I. The Role of Ascorbic Acid in Host Resistance. *Chemico-Biological Interactions* 9: 273–283.

Cameron, E.; Pauling, L. (1976) Supplemental Ascorbate in the Supportive Treatment of Cancer: I. Prolongation of Survival Times in Terminal Human Cancer. *Proceedings of the National Academy of Sciences, U.S.A.* October.

Cathcart, R. F. (1975) Clinical Trial of Vitamin C. *Medical Tribune,* June 25.

Charleston, S. S.; Clegg, K. M. (1972) Ascorbic Acid and the Common Cold. *The Lancet* 1: 1401.

Chatterjee, I. B.; Majumder, A. K.; Nandi, B. K.; Subramanian, N. (1975) Synthesis and Some Major Functions of Vitamin C in Animals. In King and Burns, eds., *Second Conference on Vitamin C.* New York Academy of Sciences, New York.

Chaudhuri, C. R.; Chatterjee, I. B. (1969) L-Ascorbic Acid Synthesis in Birds: Phylogenetic Trend. *Science* 164: 435–436.

Cheraskin, E.; Ringsdorf, W. M., Jr. (1971) *New Hope for Incurable Diseases.* Exposition Press, Jericho, New York.

Cheraskin, E.; Ringsdorf, W. M., Jr.; Brecher, A. (1974) *Psychodietetics.* Stein and Day, New York.

Chope, H. D.; Breslow, L. (1955) Nutritional Status of the Aging. *American Journal of Public Health* 46: 61–67.

Clegg, K. M.; Macdonald, J. M. (1975) L-Ascorbic Acid and D-Isoascorbic Acid in a Common Cold Survey. *The American Journal of Clinical Nutrition* 28: 973–976.

Cochrane, W. A. (1965) Overnutrition in Prenatal and Neonatal

Life: A Problem? *Journal of the Canadian Medical Association* 93: 893-899.

Collier, R. (1974) *The Plague of the Spanish Lady*. Atheneum, New York.

Committee on Animal Nutrition (1972) *Nutrient Requirements of Laboratory Animals: Cat, Guinea Pig, Hamster, Monkey, Mouse, Rat*. National Research Council, National Academy of Sciences, Washington, D. C.

Cottingham, E.; Mills, C. A. (1943) Influence of Temperature and Vitamin Deficiency Upon Phagocytic Functions. *Journal of Immunology* 47: 493–502.

Coulehan, J. L.; Reisinger, K. S.; Rogers, K. D.; Bradley, D. W. (1974) Vitamin C Prophylaxis in a Boarding School. *The New England Journal of Medicine* 290: 6–10.

Cowan, D. W.; Diehl, H. S. (1950) Antihistaminic Agents and Ascorbic Acid in the Early Treatment of the Common Cold. *Journal of the American Medical Association* 143: 421–424.

Cowan, D. W.; Diehl, H. S.; Baker, A. B. (1942) Vitamins for the Prevention of Colds. *Journal of the American Medical Association* 120: 1268–1271.

Dahlberg, G.; Engel, A.; Rydin, H. (1944) The Value of Ascorbic Acid as a Prophylactic Against Common Colds. *Acta Medica Scandinavica* 119: 540–561.

Davidson, S.; Passmore, R.; Brock, J. F.; Truswell, A. S. (1975) *Human Nutrition and Dietetics*. Churchill Livingstone, Edinburgh, London, and New York.

Debré, R. (1918) L'Anergie dans la grippe. *Comptes Rendus Soc. Biol.* (Paris) 81: 913–914.

Debré, R.; Celers, J. (1970) *Clinical Virology*. W. B. Saunders Company, Philadelphia.

DeCosse, J. J.; Adams, M. B.; Kuvma, J. F.; LoGerfo, P.; Condon, R. E. (1975) Effect of Ascorbic Acid on Rectal Polyps of Patients with Familial Polyposis. *Surgery* 78: 608–612.

Demole, V. (1934) Praktische Skorbutkost Nr. 111 aus Haferflocken und Trockenmilch. *Zeitschrift für Vitaminforschung* 3: 89–91.

Dice, J. F.; Daniel, C. W. (1973) The Hypoglycemic Effect of Ascorbic Acid in a Juvenile-onset Diabetic. *International*

Research Communications System 1: 41.

Diehl, H. S. (1970) Vitamin C and Colds. *New York Times*, December 26.

Drake, R. M.; Buechley, R. W.; Breslow, L.; Chope, H. D. (1957) A Seven-Year Following of the San Mateo Nutrition-Study Population. Presented before the Western Branch of the American Public Health Association, Long Beach, California, May 31, 1957.

Dreisbach, R. H. (1969) *Handbook of Poisoning: Diagnosis and Treatment,* 6th edition. Lange Medical Publications, Los Altos, California.

Dugal, L. P. (1961) Ascorbic Acid and Acclimatization to Cold in Monkeys. *Annals of the New York Academy of Science* 92: 307–317.

Dujarric de la Rivière, R. (1918) La Grippe est-elle une maladie à virus filtrant? *Comptes rendus Acad. Sci.* (Paris) 167: 606.

Dykes, M. H. M.; Meier, P. (1975) Ascorbic Acid and the Common Cold. *Journal of the American Medical Association* 231: 1073–1079.

Elliott, B. (1973) Ascorbic Acid: Efficacy in the Prevention of Symptoms of Respiratory Infection on a Polaris Submarine. *International Research Communications System,* May.

Enloe, C. F., Jr. (1971) The Virtue of Theory. *Nutrition Today,* Jánuary–February, p. 21.

Ericsson, Y.; Lundbeck, H. (1955) Antimicrobial Effect *in vitro* of the Ascorbic Acid Oxidation. I. Effect on Bacteria, Fungi and Viruses in Pure Cultures. II. Influence of Various Chemical and Physical Factors. *Acta Pathologica et Microbiologica Scandinavica* 37: 493–527.

Ertel, H. (1941) Der Verlauf der Vitamin C-Prophylaxen in Frühjahr. *Die Ernährung* 6: 269–273.

Fabricant, N. D.; Conklin, G. (1965) *The Dangerous Cold.* The Macmillan Company, New York.

Faulkner, J. M.; Taylor, F. H. L. (1937) Vitamin C and Infection. *Annals of Internal Medicine* 10: 146–152.

Fletcher, J. M.; Fletcher, I. C. (1951) Vitamin C and the Common Cold. *British Medical Journal* 1: 887.

Food and Nutrition Board, U.S. National Research Council (1974) *Recommended Dietary Allowances,* 8th revised edition. National Academy of Sciences Pub. 2216, National Academy of Sciences, Washington, D.C.

Francis, T., Jr. (1953) Influenza: Newe Acquayantance. (James D. Bruce Memorial Lecture). *Annals of Internal Medicine* 39: 203–221.

Franz, W. L.; Sands, G. W.; Heyl, H. L. (1956) Blood Ascorbic Acid Level in Bioflavonoid and Ascorbic Acid Therapy of Common Cold. *Journal of the American Medical Association* 162: 1224–1226.

Friedman, G. J.; Sherry, S.; Ralli, E. P. (1940) Mechanism of Excretion of Vitamin C by Human Kidney at Low and Normal Plasma Levels of Ascorbic Acid. *Journal of Clinical Investigations* 19: 685–689.

Funk, C. (1912) The Etiology of the Deficiency Diseases: Beri-Beri, Polyneuritis in Birds, Epidemic Dropsy, Scurvy, Experimental Scurvy in Animals, Infantile Scurvy, Ship Beri-Beri, Pellagra. *J. St. Med.* 20: 341–368.

Gildersleeve, D. (1967) Why Organized Medicine Sneezes at the Common Cold. *Fact,* July–August, pp. 21–23.

Ginter, E. (1970) *The Role of Ascorbic Acid in Cholesterol Metabolism.* Slovak Academy of Sciences, Bratislava.

Ginter, E. (1975) *The Role of Ascorbic Acid in Cholesterol Catabolism and Atherogenesis.* Slovak Academy of Sciences, Bratislava.

Ginter, E. (1973) Cholesterol: Vitamin C Controls Its Transformation to Bile Acids. *Science* 179: 702–704.

Glazebrook, A. J.; Thomson, S. (1942) The Administration of Vitamin C in a Large Institution and its Effect on General Health and Resistance to Infection. *Journal of Hygiene* 42: 1–19.

Gray, G. W. (1941) *The Advancing Front of Medicine.* Whittlesey House, New York.

Greenblatt, R. B. (1955) Bioflavonoids and the Capillary: Management of Habitual Abortion. *Annals of the New York Academy of Sciences* 61: 713–720.

Greenwood, J. (1964) Optimum Vitamin C Intake as a Factor in the

Preservation of Disc Integrity. *Medical Annals of the District of Columbia* 33: 274–276.

Harris, L. J.; Ray, S. N. (1935) Diagnosis of Vitamin C-Subnutrition by Urinalysis With Note on Antiscorbutic Value of Human Milk. *The Lancet* 1: 71–77.

Harris, A.; Robinson, A. B.; Pauling, L. (1973) Blood Plasma L-Ascorbic Acid Concentration for Oral L-Ascorbic Acid Dosage up to 12 Grams per Day. *International Research Communications System*, December, p. 19.

Hawkins, D.; Pauling, L. (1973) *Orthomolecular Psychiatry*. W. H. Freeman and Company, San Francisco.

Herbert, V.; Jacob, E. (1974) Destruction of Vitamin B_{12} by Ascorbic Acid. *Journal of the American Medical Association* 230: 241–242.

Herjanic, M.; Moss-Herjanic, B. L. (1967) Ascorbic Acid Test in Psychiatric Patients. *Journal of Schizophrenia* 1: 257–260.

Herz, A. (1917) Über hemorrhagische Diathese: Purpura symptomatica und Skorbut bei Typhus abdominalis, Paratyphus A und Paratyphus B. *Wiener klinische Wochenschrift* 22: 675–688.

Hindson, T. C. (1968) Ascorbic Acid for Prickly Heat. *The Lancet* 1: 1347–1348.

Hoffer, A. (1962) *Niacin Therapy in Psychiatry*. Charles C. Thomas, Springfield, Illinois.

Hoffer, A. (1971) Ascorbic Acid and Toxicity. *New England Journal of Medicine* 285: 635–636.

Hoffer, A.; Osmond, H. (1966) *How to Live With Schizophrenia*. University Books, New Hyde Park, New York.

Holmes, H. N. (1946) The Use of Vitamin C in Traumatic Shock. *Ohio State Medical Journal* 42: 1261–1264.

Hopkins, F. G. (1912) Feeding Experiments Illustrating the Importance of Accessory Factors in Normal Dietaries. *Journal of Physiology* (London) 44: 425–460.

Hume, R.; Weyers, E. (1973) Changes in Leucocyte Ascorbic Acid During the Common Cold. *Scottish Medical Journal* 18: 3–7.

Isaacs, A.; Lindenmann, J. (1957) Virus Interference. I. The Interferon. *Proceedings of the Royal Society of London* B147: 258–267.

Jaffe, R. M.; Kasten, B.; Young, D. S.; MacLowry, J. D. (1975) False-Negative Stool Occult Blood Tests Caused by Ingestion of Ascorbic Acid (Vitamin C). *Annals of Internal Medicine* 83: 824–826.

Javert, C. T.; Stander, H. J. (1943) Plasma Vitamin C and Prothrombin Concentration in Pregnancy and in Threatened, Spontaneous, and Habitual Abortion. *Surgery, Gynecology, and Obstetrics* 76: 115–122.

Johnson, G. T. (1975) *What You Should Know About Health Care Before You Call a Doctor.* McGraw-Hill Book Company, New York.

Jungeblut, C. W. (1935) Inactivation of Poliomyelitis Virus by Crystalline Vitamin C (Ascorbic Acid). *Journal of Experimental Medicine* 62: 517–521.

Karlowski, T. R.; Chalmers, T. C.; Frenkel, L. D.; Kapikian, A. Z.; Lewis, T. L.; Lynch, J. M. (1975) Ascorbic Acid for the Common Cold: A Prophylactic and Therapeutic Trial. *Journal of the American Medical Association* 231: 1038–1042.

Kimbarowski, J. A.; Mokrow, N. J. (1967) Farbige Ausfällungsreaktion des Harns nach Kimbarowski als Index der Wirkung von Ascorbinsäure bei Behandlung der Virusgrippe. *Deutsche Gesundheitswesen* 22: 2413–2418.

Klenner, F. R. (1948) Virus Pneumonia and its Treatment With Vitamin C. *Journal of Southern Medicine and Surgery* 110: 60–63.

Klenner, F. R. (1949) The Treatment of Poliomyelitis and Other Virus Diseases with Vitamin C. *Journal of Southern Medicine and Surgery* 111: 210–214.

Klenner, F. R. (1951) Massive Doses of Vitamin C and the Viral Diseases. *Journal of Southern Medicine and Surgery* 113: 101–107.

Klenner, F. R. (1971) Observations on the Dose and Administration of Ascorbic Acid When Employed Beyond the Range of a Vitamin in Human Pathology. *Journal of Applied Nutrition* 23: 61–88.

Klenner, F. R. (1974) Significance of High Daily Intake of Ascorbic

Acid in Preventive Medicine. *Journal of the International Academy of Preventive Medicine* 1: 45–69.

Klenner, F. R. (with Bartz, F. H.) (1969) *The Key to Good Health: Vitamin C.* Graphic Arts Research Foundation, Chicago, Illinois.

Kodicek, E. H.; Young, F. G. (1969) Captain Cook and Scurvy. *Notes and Records of the Royal Society of London* 24: 43–60.

Kogan, B. A. (1970) *Health.* Harcourt, Brace and World, Inc., New York.

Korbsch, R. (1938) Über die Kupierung entzündlich-allergischer Zustände durch die L-Askorbinsäure. *Medizinische Klinik* 34: 1500–1501.

Kubala, A. L.; Katz, M. M. (1960) Nutritional Factors in Psychological Test Behavior. *Journal of Genetic Psychology* 96: 343–352.

Kubler, W.; Gehler, J. (1970) Zur Kinetik der enteralen Ascorbinsäure-resorption zur Berechnung nicht dosisproportionaler Resorptionsvorgänge. *Internationale Zeitschrift für Vitaminforschung* 40: 442–453.

Kundin, W. C. (1970) Hong Kong A-2 Influenza Virus Infection Among Swine During a Human Epidemic in Taiwan. *Nature* 228: 857.

Lahann, H. (1970) *Vitamin C, Forschung und Praxis.* Merck, Darmstadt.

Lamden, M. P.; Chrystowski, G. A. (1954) Urinary Oxalate Excretion by Man Following Ascorbic Acid Ingestion. *Proceedings of the Society for Experimental Biology and Medicine* 85: 190–192.

Lunin, N. (1881) Über die Bedeutung der anorganischen Salze für die Ernährung des Tieres. *Zeitschrift für physiologische Chemie* 5:31–39.

McCormick, W. J. (1952) Ascorbic Acid as a Chemotherapeutic Agent. *Archives of Pediatrics* 69: 151–155.

Macon, W. L. (1956) Citrus Bioflavonoids in the Treatment of the Common Cold. *Industrial Medicine and Surgery* 25: 525–527.

Marckwell, N. W. (1947) Vitamin C in the Prevention of Colds. *Medical Journal of Australia* 2: 777–778.

Masek, J.; Neradilova, M.; Hejda, S. (1972) Vitamin C and Respiratory Infections. *Review of Czechoslovak Medicine* 18: 228–235.

Matsuo, E.; Skinsnes, O. K.; Chang, P. H. C. (1975) Acid Mucopolysaccharide Metabolism in Leprosy. III. Hyaluronic Acid Mycobacterial Growth Enhancement, and Growth Suppression by Saccharic Acid and Vitamin C as Inhibitors of Betaglucuronidase. *International Journal of Leprosy* 43: 1–13.

Miller, T. E. (1969) Killing and Lysis of Gram-Negative Bacteria Through the Synergistic Effect of Hydrogen Peroxide, Ascorbic Acid, and Lysozyme. *Journal of Bacteriology* 98: 949–955.

Murata, A. (1975) Virucidal Activity of Vitamin C: Vitamin C for Prevention and Treatment of Viral Diseases. *Proceedings of the First Intersectional Congress of Microbiological Societies,* Science Council of Japan 3: 432–442.

Murata, A.; Kitagawa, K. (1973) Mechanism of Inactivation of Bacteriophage J1 by Ascorbic Acid. *Agricultural and Biological Chemistry* 37: 1145–1151.

Murata, A.; Kitagawa, K.; Saruno, R. (1971) Inactivation of Bacteriophages by Ascorbic Acid. *Agricultural and Biological Chemistry* 35: 294–296.

Newmark, H. L.; Scheiner, J.; Marcus, M.; Prabhudesai, M. (1976) Stability of Vitamin B_{12} in the Presence of Ascorbic Acid. *The American Journal of Clinical Nutrition* 29: 645–649.

Nicolé, C.; LeBailly, C. (1918) Quelque notions expérimentales sur le virus de la grippe. *Comptes rendus Acad. Sci.* (Paris) 167: 607–610.

Omura, H.; Fukumoto, Y.; Tomita, Y.; Shinohara, K. (1975) Action of 5-Methyl-3,4-dihydroxytetrone on Deoxyribonucleic Acid. *Journal of the Faculty of Agriculture, Kyushu University,* 19: 139–148.

Omura, H.; Tomita, Y.; Nakamura, Y.; Murakami, H. (1974) Antitumoric Potentiality of Some Ascorbate Derivatives. *Journal of the Faculty of Agriculture, Kyushu University,* 18: 181–189.

Paeschke, K. D.; Vasterling, H. W. (1968) Photometrischer Ascorbinsäure-Test zur Bestimmung der Ovulation, verglichen mit anderen Methoden der Ovulationsterminbestimmung. *Zen-*

tralblatt für Gynäkologie 90: 817–820.

Passmore, R. (1971) That man. . . . Pauling! *Nutrition Today,* January–February, pp. 17–18.

Passwater, R. A. (1975) *Supernutrition.* The Dial Press, New York.

Paul, J. H.; Freese, H. L. (1933) An Epidemiological and Bacteriological Study of the "Common Cold" in an Isolated Arctic Community (Spitsbergen). *American Journal of Hygiene* 17: 517–535.

Pauling, L. (1968a) Orthomolecular Psychiatry. *Science* 160: 265–271.

Pauling, L. (1968b) Orthomolecular Somatic and Psychiatric Medicine. *Journal of Vital Substances and Diseases of Civilization* 14: 1–3.

Pauling, L. (1970a) *Vitamin C and the Common Cold.* W. H. Freeman and Company, San Francisco.

Pauling, L. (1970b) Evolution and the Need for Ascorbic Acid. *Proceedings of the National Academy of Sciences, U.S.A.* 67: 1643–1648.

Pauling, L. (1971a) *Vitamin C and the Common Cold,* revised edition. Bantam Books, New York.

Pauling, L. (1971b) That man. . . . Pauling! *Nutrition Today,* March–April, pp. 21–24.

Pauling, L. (1971c) Vitamin C and the Common Cold. *Journal of the American Medical Association* 216: 332.

Pauling, L. (1971d) Vitamin C and Colds. *New York Times,* January 17.

Pauling, L. (1973a) Preventive Nutrition. *Medicine on the Midway* 27: 15–17.

Pauling, L. (1973b) *Vitamin C and the Common Cold,* abridged edition. Bantam Books, New York.

Pauling, L. (1974a) Early Evidence About Vitamin C and the Common Cold. *Journal of Orthomolecular Psychiatry* 3: 139–151.

Pauling, L. (1974b) On the Orthomolecular Environment of the Mind: Orthomolecular Theory. *American Journal of Psychiatry* 131: 1251–1257.

Pauling, L. (1974c) Are Recommended Daily Allowances for Vitamin C Adequate? *Proceedings of the National Academy of Sciences, U.S.A.* 71: 4442–4446.

Pauling, L. (1976a) On Fighting Swine Flu. *New York Times,* June 5.

Pauling, L. (1976b) Ascorbic Acid and the Common Cold: Evaluation of its Efficacy and Toxicity. *Medical Tribune,* March 24.

Pauling, L. (1976c) The Case for Vitamin C in Maintaining Health and Preventing Disease. *Modern Medicine,* July, pp. 68–72.

Portman, O. W.; Alexander, M.; Maruffo, C. A.; (1967) Nutritional Control of Arterial Lipid Composition in Squirrel Monkeys. *Journal of Nutrition* 91: 35–44.

Régnier, E. (1968) The Administration of Large Doses of Ascorbic Acid in the Prevention and Treatment of the Common Cold, Parts I and II. *Review of Allergy* 22: 835–846, 948–956.

Renker, K.; Wegner, S. (1954) Vitamin C-Prophylaxe in der Volkswerft Stralsund. *Deutsche Gesundheitswesen* 9: 702–706.

Rinehart, J. F.; Greenberg, L. D. (1956) Vitamin B_6 Deficiency in the Rhesus Monkey With Particular Reference to the Occurrence of Atherosclerosis, Dental Caries, and Hepatic Cirrhosis. *American Journal of Clinical Nutrition* 4: 318–327.

Ritzel, G. (1961) *Kritische Beurteilung des Vitamins C als Prophylacticum und Therapeuticum der Erkältungskrankheiten. Helvetica Medica Acta* 28: 63–68.

Rosenberg, H.; Feldzamen, A. N. (1974) *The Doctor's Book of Vitamin Therapy.* G. P. Putnam's Sons, New York.

Ross, W. S. (1971) Vitamin C: Does It Really Help? *Readers Digest* 98: 129–132.

Ruskin, S. L. (1938) Calcium Cevitamate (Calcium Ascorbate) in the Treatment of Acute Rhinitis. *Annals of Otology, Rhinology, and Laryngology* 47: 502–511.

Sabiston, B. H.; Radomski, N. W. (1974) Health Problems and Vitamin C in Canadian Northern Military Operations. *Defence and Civil Institute of Environmental Medicine Report No. 7 4-R-1012.*

Salomon, L. L.; Stubbs, D. W. (1961) Some Aspects of the Metabolism of Ascorbic Acid in Rats. *Annals of the New York Academy of Sciences* 92: 128–140.

Samborskaya, E. P.; Ferdman, T. D. (1966) The Problem of the Mechanism of Artificial Abortion by Use of Ascorbic Acid. *Bjulletin Eksperimentalnoi Biologii i Meditsinii* 62: 96–98.

Scheunert, A. (1949) Der Tagesbedarf des Erwachsenen an Vitamin C. *Internationale Zeitschrift für Vitaminforschung* 20: 371–386.

Schlegel, J. U.; Pipkin, G. E.; Nishimura, R.; Schultz, G. N. (1970) The Role of Ascorbic Acid in the Prevention of Bladder Tumor Formation. *Journal of Urology* 103: 155–159.

Schmeck, H. M. Jr. (1973) Research Funds and Disease Effects Held Out of Step. *New York Times*, February 10.

Schwartz, P. L. (1970) Ascorbic Acid in Wound Healing—A Review. *Journal of the American Dietetic Association* 56: 497–503.

Schwerdt, P. R.; Schwerdt, C. E. (1975) Effect of Ascorbic Acid on Rhinovirus Replication in WI-38 Cells. *Proceedings of the Society for Experimental Biology and Medicine* 148: 1237–1243.

Selter, M. (1918) Zur Aetiologie der Influenza. *Deutsche medizinische Wochenschrift,* 44, 932–933.

Skinsnes, O. K.; Matsuo, E. (1976) Acid Mucopolysaccharide Metabolism Related to Leprosy Susceptibility. Preprint.

Smith, J. W. G.; Fletcher, W. B.; Wherry, P. J. (1975) Reactions to Injected Influenza Vaccine. *Development of Biological Standards* 28: 377–388.

Smith, W., Andrewes; C. H.; Laidlow, P. (1933) A Virus Obtained From Influenza Patients. *The Lancet* 225: 66–68.

Sokoloff, B.; Hori, M.; Saelhof, C. C.; Wrzolek, T.; Imai, T. (1966) Aging, Atherosclerosis, and Ascorbic Acid Metabolism. *Journal of the American Geriatric Society* 14: 1239–1260.

Spero, L. M.; Anderson, T. W. (1973) Ascorbic Acid and Common Colds. *British Medical Journal* 4: 354.

Spittle, C. R. (1971) Atherosclerosis and Vitamin C. *The Lancet* 2: 1280–1281.

Stare, F. J. (1969) *Eating for Good Health.* Cornerstone Library, New York.

Stone, I. (1965) Studies of a Mammalian Enzyme System for Producing Evolutionary Evidence on Man. *American Journal of*

Physical Anthropology 23: 83–86.

Stone, I. (1966a) On the Genetic Etiology of Scurvy. *Acta Geneticae Medicae et Gemellologiae* 15: 345–349.

Stone, I. (1966b) Hypoascorbemia: The Genetic Disease Causing the Human Requirement for Exogenous Ascorbic Acid. *Perspectives in Biology and Medicine* 10: 133–134.

Stone, I. (1967) The Genetic Disease Hypoascorbemia. *Acta Geneticae Medicae et Gemellologiae* 16: 52–60.

Stone, I. (1972) *The Healing Factor: Vitamin C Against Disease.* Grosset and Dunlap, New York.

Stuart-Harris, C. (1976) Swine Influenza Virus in Man: Zoonosis or Human Pandemic? *The Lancet* 2: 31–32.

Subcommittee on Laboratory Animal Nutrition (1972) *Nutrient Requirements of Laboratory Animals,* 2nd edition. National Academy of Sciences, Washington, D.C.

Szent-Györgyi, A. (1933) Identification of Vitamin C. *Nature* 131: 225–226.

Szent-Györgyi, A. (1937) *Studies on Biological Oxidation and Some of Its Catalysts,* Szeged, Hungary.

Tebrock, H. E.; Arminio, J. J.; Johnston, J. H. (1956) Usefulness of Bioflavonoids and Ascorbic Acid in Treatment of Common Cold. *Journal of the American Medical Association* 162: 1227–1233.

Thaddea, S.; Hoffmeister, W. (1937) Die Bedeutung des C-Vitamins für Infektionsablauf und Krankheitsabwehr. *Zeitschrift für klinische Medizin* 132: 379–416.

VanderKamp, H. (1966) A Biochemical Abnormality in Schizophrenia Involving Ascorbic Acid. *International Journal of Neurochemistry and Psychiatry* 2: 204–206.

Vargus Magne, R. (1963) Vitamin C in Treatment of Influenza. *El Dia Medico* 35: 1714–1715.

Virno, M.; Bucci, M. G.; Pecori-Giraldi, J.; Missiroli, A. (1967) Oral Treatment of Glaucoma With Vitamin C. *The Eye, Ear, Nose, and Throat Monthly* 46: 1502–1508.

Wagner, A. F.; Folkers, K. (1964) *Vitamins and Coenzymes.* Interscience Publishers, New York.

Walker, G. H.; Bynoe, M. L.; Tyrrell, D. A. J. (1967) Trial of Ascorbic Acid in Prevention of Colds. *British Medical Journal* 1: 603–606.

Waugh, W. A.; King, C. G. (1932) Isolation and Identification of Vitamin C. *Journal of Biological Chemistry* 97: 325–331.

Whelan, E.; Stare, F. J. (1975) *Panic in the Pantry*. Atheneum, New York.

White, P. L. (1975) Editorial: Megavitamin This and Megavitamin That. *Journal of the American Medical Association* 233: 538–539.

Williams, R. J. (1967) *You Are Extraordinary*. Random House, New York.

Williams, R. J. (1973) *Biochemical Individuality*. University of Texas Press, Austin.

Williams, R. J. (1975) *Physician's Handbook of Nutritional Science*. Charles C. Thomas, Springfield, Illinois.

Williams, R. J.; Deason, G. (1967) Individuality In Vitamin C Needs. *Proceedings of the National Academy of Sciences U.S.A.* 57: 1638–1641.

Willis, G. C.; Fishman, S. (1955) Ascorbic Acid Content of Human Arterial Tissue. *Canadian Medical Association Journal* 72: 500–503.

Wilson, C. W. M. (1967) Ascorbic Acid and Colds. *British Medical Journal* 2: 698–699.

Wilson, C. W. M.; Loh, H. S. (1970) Ascorbic Acid and Upper Respiratory Inflammation. *Acta Allergologica* 24: 367–370.

Wilson, C. W.; Loh, H. S. (1973) Vitamin C and Colds. *The Lancet* 1: 1058–1059.

Wilson, C. W.; Loh, H. S.; Foster, F. G. (1976a) The Beneficial Effect of Vitamin C on the Common Cold. *European Journal of Clinical Pharmacology* 6: 26–32.

Wilson, C. W.; Loh, H. S.; Foster, F. G. (1976b) Common Cold Symptomatology and Vitamin C. *European Journal of Clinical Pharmacology* 6: 196–202.

Winitz, M.; Graff, J.; Seedman, D. A. (1964) Effect of Dietary Carbohydrate on Serum Cholesterol Levels. *Archives of Biochemistry and Biophysics* 108: 576–579.

Winitz, M.; Seedman, D. A.; Graff, J. (1970) Studies in Metabolic Nutrition Employing Chemically Defined Diets. I. Extended Feeding of Normal Adult Males. *American Journal of Clinical Nutrition* 23: 525–546.

Wohl, M. G.; Goodhart, R. S., Eds. (1968) *Modern Nutrition in Health and Disease,* 4th edition. Lea and Febiger, Philadelphia.

Wolfer, J. A.; Farmer, C. J.; Carroll, W. W.; Manshardt, D. O. (1947) An Experimental Study in Wound Healing in Vitamin-C Depleted Human Subjects. *Surgery, Gynecology, and Obstetrics* 84: 1–15.

Yandell, H. R. (1951) The Treatment of Extensive Burns. *American Surgeon* 17: 351–360.

Yew, M. S. (1973) "Recommended Daily Allowances" for Vitamin C. *Proceedings of the National Academy of Sciences, U.S.A.* 70: 969–972.

Yonemoto, R. H.; Chretien, P. B.; Fehniger, T. F. (1976) Enhanced Lymphocyte Blastogenesis by Oral Ascorbic Acid. *American Society of Clinical Oncologists,* p. 288.

Yudkin, J. (1972) *Sweet and Dangerous.* Peter H. Wyden, Inc., New York.

Zamenhof, S.; Eichhorn, H. H. (1967) Study of Microbial Evolution Through Loss of Biosynthetic Functions: Establishment of "Defective" Mutants. *Nature* 216: 456–458.

Zuckerkandl, E.; Pauling, L. (1962) Molecular Disease, Evolution, and Genic Heterogeneity, in Kasha, M., and Pullman, b., Eds., *Horizons in Biochemistry* (Szent-Györgyi Dedicatory Volume), Academic Press, New York, p. 189.

Indexes

NAME INDEX

SUBJECT INDEX

ABOUT THE AUTHOR

Linus Pauling was born in Portland, Oregon, on 28 February 1901.
His father was a druggist who died when Linus was nine years old.
Linus worked his way through the Oregon Agricultural College in
Corvallis, where he majored in chemical engineering. As an under-
graduate he showed great promise and helped to support himself by
teaching chemistry. Because of his financial responsibility for his
mother and two younger sisters, he dropped out of his college studies
for one year and worked as a full-time teaching assistant in the
quantitative analysis courses. (He first met his future wife, Ava Helen
Miller, when she was a student in a chemistry course that he taught.)
During the summers he worked at a variety of jobs, mainly as a
paving-plant inspector.

After receiving his degree in 1922, he earned his doctorate at the
California Institute of Technology in 1925, then went on to eighteen
months of study in Munich, Zurich, and Copenhagen. He returned to
the California Institute of Technology as a member of the faculty,
and he remained there until 1964. After several years in the Center
for the Study of Democratic Institutions in Santa Barbara, California,
the University of California, San Diego, and Stanford University, he
became Research Professor in the Linus Pauling Institute of Science
and Medicine, Menlo Park, California.

Linus Pauling has long been deeply concerned with the alleviation
of human suffering, and he has brought his scientific knowledge to

bear on such problems as the causes of genetic mutation, the transmission of aberrant genes, and the deleterious effects of protein molecules with abnormal structure. On occasions, his views have led him to take strong public positions—some decidedly unpopular or unpolitic—against cigarette smoking, against the maintenance of preventable hereditary diseases in human populations, against the testing, proliferation and use of atomic and nuclear weapons, and against war in general.

His achievements in science, medicine, and the promotion of human welfare have brought him countless honors, such as the Phillips Medal of the American College of Physicians for his contributions to internal medicine, the Gold Medal of the French Academy of Medicine, the Baxter Award in anesthesiology, the Rudolf Virchow Medal, the Thomas Addis Medal of the American Nephrosis Foundation, the *Modern Medicine* Award, the Humanist of the Year Award, and many others, including dozens of honorary degrees and election to honorary membership in twenty scientific societies in twelve countries. Linus Pauling has been awarded two Nobel Prizes: the 1954 Nobel Prize for Chemistry and the 1962 Nobel Prize for Peace.

His principal research at present is on the molecular basis of disease, including mental disease. He has published more than four hundred papers, most of which present the results of original investigations, and he is the author of a number of influential books, including *Introduction to Quantum Mechanics* (with E. B. Wilson, Jr.), *The Nature of the Chemical Bond, General Chemistry, College Chemistry, The Architecture of Molecules* (with Roger Hayward), and *No More War!*. His 1970 book *Vitamin C and the Common Cold* was given the Phi Beta Kappa award as the best scientific book of the year.